ETHICAL
PRACTICE
IN
GEROPSYCHOLOGY

ETHICAL PRACTICE IN GEROPSYCHOLOGY

Shane S. Bush, Rebecca S. Allen, and Victor A. Molinari

American Psychological Association • Washington, DC

Published by
American Psychological Association
750 First Street, NE
Washington, DC 20002
www.apa.org

To order
APA Order Department
P.O. Box 92984
Washington, DC 20090-2984
Tel: (800) 374-2721; Direct: (202) 336-5510
Fax: (202) 336-5502; TDD/TTY: (202) 336-6123
Online: www.apa.org/pubs/books
E-mail: order@apa.org

In the U.K., Europe, Africa, and the Middle East, copies may be ordered from
American Psychological Association
3 Henrietta Street
Covent Garden, London
WC2E 8LU England

Typeset in Goudy by Circle Graphics, Inc., Columbia, MD

Printer: Bang Printing, Brainerd, MI
Cover Designer: FALCONE Creative Services, Potomac, MD

The opinions and statements published are the responsibility of the authors, and such opinions and statements do not necessarily represent the policies of the American Psychological Association.

Library of Congress Cataloging-in-Publication Data

Names: Bush, Shane S., 1965- author. | Allen, Rebecca S., author. | Molinari, Victor, 1952- author.
Title: Ethical practice in geropsychology / Shane S. Bush, Rebecca S. Allen, and Victor A. Molinari.
Description: Washington, DC : American Psychological Association, [2017] | Includes bibliographical references and index.
Identifiers: LCCN 2016025240 | ISBN 9781433826269 | ISBN 1433826267
Subjects: LCSH: Geriatric psychiatry—Moral and ethical aspects. | Older people—Mental health services—Moral and ethical aspects. | Older people—Psychology. | Clinical psychology—Moral and ethical aspects.
Classification: LCC RC451.4.A5 B837 2017 | DDC 618.97/689—dc23 LC record available at https://lccn.loc.gov/2016025240

British Library Cataloguing-in-Publication Data
A CIP record is available from the British Library.

Printed in the United States of America
First Edition

http://dx.doi.org/10.1037/0000010-000

To our mentors, clients, and students—those from whom
we have learned most of what we know about
ethical practice in geropsychology.

IMPORTANT NOTICE

CONTENTS

ACKNOWLEDGMENTS

Many colleagues, too numerous to name, have contributed to the current understanding of ethical issues in geropsychology. We are grateful to those who have added to this important, although sometimes underappreciated, body of knowledge. It is through their earlier efforts that we were able to bring together the concepts presented in this book. We are also very thankful to Susan Reynolds, senior acquisitions editor at APA Books, for her enthusiasm about the idea for this book and her support in bringing it to fruition. Most of all, we are grateful to the older adults who allow us to work with them during some of the most meaningful and trying times of their lives in ways that we find personally and professionally rewarding.

ETHICAL PRACTICE
IN
GEROPSYCHOLOGY

INTRODUCTION

The aging of the U.S. population is well-established, and psychologists are playing an increasingly prominent role in the care and well-being of older adults. The emergence of geropsychology as a subspecialty area of clinical practice is one of the most exciting developments in psychology during the past 25 years. This development is an important step in addressing the well-established shortage of geriatric mental health practitioners (American Psychological Association [APA], 2014c; Institute of Medicine, 2012). Between 5.6 million and 8 million older Americans have one or more mental health disorders. Because the number of adults age 65 and older is projected to rise from 40.3 million in 2010 to 72.1 million in 2030, the aging of America has profound implications for psychology and health care in general. Unfortunately, the number of psychologists working in or entering practice with older adults is disconcertingly small, and those who are competent to manage complex older adult cases are in short supply (Institute of

http://dx.doi.org/10.1037/0000010-001
Ethical Practice in Geropsychology, by S. S. Bush, R. S. Allen, and V. A. Molinari

Medicine, 2012). Thus, geropsychology is still an underrepresented area of practice. Providing clinical services to older adults presents challenges that may be novel for those trained to work with younger adults. The following vignette illustrates some common issues a psychologist might encounter with an older client.[1]

After suffering a recent stroke, Mrs. Jones presented with her daughter to the interdisciplinary primary care clinic in geriatric medicine at the local university teaching hospital. The daughter had made the appointment for Mrs. Jones because she was concerned about her mother's mental capacity for making decisions about important life issues, including living independently. Mrs. Jones and her daughter had a difference of opinion regarding the safety of Mrs. Jones's current living situation; they shared their concerns with the geropsychologists and other members of the geriatric care team, which included a geriatrician, nurse, pharmacist, and psychology and social work trainees. Mrs. Jones clearly and emphatically stated her preference for continuing to live in her home of 56 years, the home that she had shared with her late husband and currently shares with four cats and one dog. Her daughter, in contrast, offered that Mrs. Jones and one cat and the dog could live in the "granny flat" recently built onto her own house roughly 70 miles away.

How might the geropsychologist approach such a situation? What additional information does the geropsychologist need? What potential ethical and legal issues may arise in working with Mrs. Jones?

The primary goal of this book is to promote the development and maintenance of ethical competence in psychology trainees and practitioners working with older adults. To achieve this goal, we present common ethical and legal issues confronting geropsychologists and illustrate ways to identify and negotiate ethical issues and challenges through the use of vignettes covering a variety of practice contexts. By increasing awareness of such issues, psychologists may choose courses of behavior that are consistent with ethical practice, thereby promoting patient care and avoiding ethical misconduct. The book draws heavily from principle-based ethics (Beauchamp & Childress, 2013) and positive ethics (Knapp & VandeCreek, 2006, 2012) in the practical application of the *Ethical Principles of Psychologists and Code of Conduct* (hereinafter referred to as the Ethics Code; APA, 2010) and related professional guidelines and resources to geropsychology.

---

[1]Proper steps were taken to protect the confidentiality of all individuals mentioned in the case examples throughout this book.

THE HISTORY OF GEROPSYCHOLOGY

Psychology as a discipline dates to the 19th century, when Wilhelm Wundt founded the first psychological research laboratory in Leipzig in 1879 and Francis Galton collected reaction time data at the first large health exhibit in London in 1884 (Birren & Schroots, 2001). APA was founded in 1892 with 31 members and G. Stanley Hall as its first president. According to Birren and Schroots (2001), however, 1950 may arbitrarily delineate the beginnings of organized university research and education in geropsychology. The Gerontological Society of America was founded in 1946, and Division 20 (Adult Development and Aging) of APA was founded in 1947.

Perhaps the strongest demarcation of the rise of clinical practice focused on the issues of aging was the establishment of the Society of Clinical Geropsychology, Division 12 Section II of APA in 1993. More recently, geropsychology was recognized as a specialty area by APA in 2011, and as of December 2014 those competent in geropsychology can now be certified by the American Board of Professional Psychology. Individuals seeking to be board certified in geropsychology must demonstrate adequate training and competence in foundational (theoretical and empirical) and functional (assessment, intervention, consultation) knowledge and skills relevant for the ethical practice of geropsychology.

The maturing of professions and specialties is reflected in the need for, and development of, guidelines, based on shared values and ideas about appropriate professional behavior, that guide members of the profession in their decisions about professional activities. With the APA (2010) Ethics Code as one primary resource, geropsychology scholars, informed by general bioethical principles, have generated additional professional guidelines that advise practitioners on best practices in geropsychology. Overviews of the application of professional ethics to geropsychology have also been published (see, e.g., Bush, 2012; Hays & Jennings, 2015; Karel, 2011), as have many articles and chapters on the ethical issues of specific aspects of practice and research with older adults. Reviewing, synthesizing, and extending these prior scholarly works on ethical practice in geropsychology in one volume marks another step in the maturation of the specialty. Although books on closely related topics such as ethical issues in geriatric mental health (Bush, 2009; Mezey et al., 2002) have been published previously, we identified the need for an ethics book specific to psychological practice with older adults to help practitioners identify ethical issues, recognize challenges, and promote ethical practice specifically from a psychological perspective that is informed by psychological ethics and resources.

The Pikes Peak model for training in geropsychology presented aspirational guidelines for the competent practice of geropsychology (Knight et al.,

2009), and Karel and colleagues (Karel, Emery, Molinari, & the CoPGTP Task Force on the Assessment of Geropsychology Competencies, 2010) used the Pikes Peak model to develop a self-assessment tool for determining practitioner competencies in assessment, intervention, consultation, research, supervision training, and management administration. Four broad aspects of training underlie this model and define geropsychology as a distinctive practice area: (a) knowledge of life span developmental theory; (b) knowledge of and skills relevant to late-life psychopathologies including dementia; (c) knowledge of medical comorbidities; and (d) knowledge of age-specific environmental contexts, including family, residential, health care, and community systems. Molinari (2012) provided further detailed suggestions for meeting the knowledge- and skills-based competencies delineated in the Pikes Peak training model by presenting tables that outline the content of the behavioral anchors of the competencies. Professional competence provides the foundation for ethical practice in geropsychology, and competence in ethical and legal aspects of practice is a component of such competent practice. That is, knowledge of ethical and legal aspects of practice is a core competency in geropsychology. Effective practice of geropsychology requires knowledge and understanding of the ethical and legal issues and challenges commonly encountered when working with older adults. Thus, geropsychology competence and ethical competence are inextricably linked.

UNIQUE ISSUES IN GEROPSYCHOLOGICAL PRACTICE

As reflected in the opening vignette, psychologists who work with older adults must address a host of unique issues not encountered with younger clients. The differences in presenting problems, involvement of others, clinical settings, and referral questions have ethical and legal implications for practitioners.

Presenting Problems

Many psychiatric disorders have a higher prevalence in later life (e.g., dementias), and some psychopathologies that occur throughout adulthood (e.g., depression, anxiety, substance abuse, psychotic symptoms) manifest in different ways or emerge for different reasons with older adults (Knight et al., 2009). Chronic medical problems are more common in late life and often are comorbid with emotional difficulties. Medications can have adverse cognitive, psychological, or behavioral effects that require the attention of geropsychologists, and polypharmacy is more frequently a problem for older adults. Loss is a common theme in late life and can be experienced in many ways, such as the loss of one's physical abilities, professional identity and finances, family members and social supports, and independence. Such losses often negatively affect psychological functioning. However, in contrast to difficulties and disorders, health promotion has garnered relatively less attention but is becoming an increasingly important area of research interest in older adults even for those who have no disorders, and geropsychologists play an important role in fostering physical and emotional well-being.

Involved Parties and Unique Settings

The involvement of family members (typically spouses or adult children) and other caregivers in psychological assessment and treatment is more common with older adults than younger adults. Such involvement can be essential, but it can also pose unique challenges for patients, families, and clinicians. Geropsychologists are likely to confront competing expectations from the consumers of services, including patients, their families or caregivers, other health care professionals, and the institutions in which many older adults are evaluated and treated. Successfully negotiating conflicting interests and expectations is required to meet the needs of patients and other stakeholders and for competent professional practice.

Treatment of older adults occurs in a wide range of settings, including the same settings as with younger adults. Older adults are also more commonly evaluated and treated in their homes, rehabilitation settings, long-term care settings, and palliative care contexts. Care providers serve older adults through education, recommendations, environmental management, and support services; helping them do so is often an important role for geropsychologists. Geropsychologists also often work closely with interdisciplinary teams, which include the patients, families, care providers, and clergy, sometimes at the request of the institutions in which older adults are receiving care. Understanding the ethical issues that emerge in such contexts promotes quality care.

Referral Questions and Services

Geropsychologists have the knowledge and skills needed to assess and address cognitive, emotional, behavioral, and social problems experienced by older adults and those involved in the lives of older adults, such as family members or other care providers. Geropsychologists provide numerous services, including individual, couples, and family treatment; group therapy; behavior management consultation; environmental design; safety recommendations; staff education; and a variety of related services. Each of the issues addressed and services provided offer opportunities for both ethical missteps and sound ethical decision-making.

FORMAT AND VIGNETTES

Part I of the book provides an overview of foundational competencies in geropsychology, with an emphasis on ethical issues and decision making. This section provides a review of the integration of psychology and geropsychology, covers the establishment and maintenance of professional competence in geropsychology, describes common ethical issues and challenges in geropsychology, and presents an ethical decision-making model to assist geropsychologists in the prevention and successful resolution of ethical dilemmas. Applying the model to each case is likely to help achieve good outcomes. When a working knowledge of the model has been achieved, the individual steps can often be addressed implicitly under conceptually integrated categories. For the cases presented in this book, we often collapse steps in the model for a more fluid discussion of the salient issues. The importance of striving to understand individual, cultural, and cohort differences is considered an essential aspect of ethical decision making and is relevant across cases and settings.

Part II covers the ethical issues often associated with the undertaking of the functional competencies expected of geropsychologists. Separate chapters address geropsychology competencies in assessment; intervention; consultation, administration, and business aspects of practice; education, training, and research; and advocacy. Vignettes present ethical issues and challenges commonly encountered in various practice settings. An attempt was made to select settings that are either more commonly encountered in the treatment of older adults compared to younger populations or are becoming increasingly important practice settings for geropsychologists. We hope that the approach used to identify ethical issues, challenges, and solutions in the contexts described will transfer to the many other practice contexts in which geropsychologists provide services that are not directly addressed herein.

For each chapter, we provide an overview of the competency, identify the professional tasks that reflect competent behavior in this domain, and provide representative examples to illustrate the ethical issues and tensions being covered. For example, the clinical and ethical tension that often emerges from the clinician's desire to both promote patient autonomy (e.g., ability to continue living independently) and maximize patient safety (e.g., recommend placement in a supervised living setting because of significant cognitive deficits) is a primary tension encountered by geropsychologists that must be anticipated, understood, and addressed. The vignettes in this book demonstrate the practical application of ethical principles and professional guidelines across a wide spectrum of geropsychology contexts. They are fictitious cases based on our combined experiences and are designed to provide a broad sample of the types of ethical issues and challenges geropsychologists experience. It is understood that the specific details of geropsychological practice can vary across the types of settings in which services are provided and across rural–urban or geographic regions of the country; thus, some aspects of the vignettes may seem atypical to readers as a result of such differences. Such details are typically less important than the underlying principles being presented. Because several good solutions to ethical challenges might be identified, we expect readers to identify different decisions that could have been made or varied courses of action that could be taken. Each vignette highlights only certain principles, although others may well be operative. We hope that the vignettes will stimulate thought and discussion.

IMPORTANT TERMINOLOGY

The Ethics Code comprises the Introduction and Applicability section, the Preamble, five General Principles, 10 Ethical Standards, and the 2010 Amendments. All references to the Ethics Code throughout the book refer to the 2010 APA Ethics Code unless otherwise specified. References to principles from other resources are accompanied by citations for the resources being referenced.

Older adults are referred to by different terms depending on the settings in which services are provided. For example, in skilled nursing facilities, the term *resident* is often used; in acute medical settings, the term *patient* is commonly used; and in private practice contexts, older adults may be referred to as *clients*. Similarly, the terms *inmate*, *litigant*, *defendant*, *plaintiff*, and *insured* are commonly used in forensic contexts. The term *client* is sometimes employed when services are provided to an individual involved in the older adult's life, such as a family member, and when services are provided to institutions or have been retained by an attorney. Rather than selecting one term and attempting to use it throughout the book, we use the term that seems most applicable to the issue being covered or the vignette being presented, with an understanding that others may prefer different terms. Additionally, unless otherwise specified, the term *geropsychologist* as used throughout the book is defined broadly to include all psychologists who provide clinical, research, teaching, supervision, or administrative services to older adults, their families, or the institutions that serve older adults. Similarly, the term *geropsychology trainee* refers to all psychology trainees who provide services to older adults.

NOTE REGARDING BOARD CERTIFICATION

Board certification in geropsychology through the American Board of Professional Psychology (ABGERO) involves a formal peer review of foundational and functional competencies in geropsychology. Examination of candidates' knowledge of ethical issues and ability to apply that knowledge to clinical cases is an important part of the examination process. We believe that a thorough understanding of the principles discussed in this book will be helpful to ABGERO candidates regarding their description of the details of the ethics materials they submit and their examination of ethical dilemmas in the vignettes presented to them. However, the book is not intended to be an ABGERO exam preparation manual, even though the issues and principles presented in this book may help geropsychologists prepare for the ethics portion of the ABGERO board certification examination.

I

FOUNDATIONAL
COMPETENCIES

1

INTEGRATING PSYCHOLOGY AND GERONTOLOGY

Life can only be understood backwards; but it must be lived forwards.
—Søren Kierkegaard

Understanding the integration of psychology and gerontology and applying that understanding in the services provided to older adults underlies competent practice of geropsychology. The purposes of this chapter are (a) to provide an overview of developmental theory; (b) to describe primary geropsychology subspecialties and work settings; (c) to describe the roles of geropsychology in interdisciplinary teams; and (d) to review the importance of understanding individual, cultural, and cohort differences when providing psychological services to older adults. The ethical practice of geropsychology requires a working knowledge of these issues.

DEVELOPMENTAL THEORY

An understanding of the ethical issues underlying geropsychology practice would be incomplete without foundational competence in life span developmental theory. Some models of adult development and aging have

http://dx.doi.org/10.1037/0000010-002
Ethical Practice in Geropsychology, by S. S. Bush, R. S. Allen, and V. A. Molinari

been proposed to help clinicians understand their older adult patients (see Whitbourne & Whitbourne, 2014, for a review). Developmental science reveals that changes throughout life result from both nature and nurture. Several models of development, including biological, psychological, sociocultural, and individual–environment interaction, describe aspects of the aging process; a biopsychosocial approach to understanding older adults reflects awareness of the various influences on adult development and aging.

Birren and Schroots (2001) noted that theoretical and empirical development of geropsychology as a discipline lagged significantly behind focus on childhood development. The first theorist to describe stages of development beyond adolescence was Erik Erikson (1950). Stages 6, 7, and 8 of his stage theory describe key developmental conflicts of young adulthood, midlife, and advanced age, respectively (Crain, 2011). According to Erikson, the positive and negative poles of each stage must be experienced and the challenges resolved, resulting in a core ego strength that would be available to the individual as a coping resource in the next phase of life. During young adulthood (referred to in Erikson's theory as Stage 6, Intimacy and Solidarity versus Isolation), the individual begins to form intimate relationships that entail effective resolution of conflict and the development of the core ego strength of love.

In Stage 7, adults at midlife experience and attempt to resolve a conflict between generativity and self-absorption, during which individuals either develop the ego strength to care for the next generation (e.g., raising children, finding ways to pass on wisdom to protégés) or fall into nonproductive self-focus. Although the popular media has characterized this struggle as a "midlife crisis," most theorists (e.g., Chiriboga, 1997; Wethington, 2000) have debunked the notion of crisis as an inevitable stage of life. Wethington (2000) reported that 26% of adults, both men and women, reported having a self-defined "midlife crisis" that might occur before age 40 or after age 50. Typical definitions for the midlife crisis provided by the middle-aged adult sample included awareness of aging, life review, change in personal approach to life, and events or transitions in family or one's job or health. The geropsychologist's understanding of individual motivation and emotional functioning at midlife often is critical to quality care later in life, consistent with Principle E (Respect for People's Rights and Dignity).

In Stage 8, Erikson (1950) proposed that as older adults begin to contemplate their own deaths, they face the developmental crisis of ego integrity versus despair. By engaging in a process of life review (Butler, 1963), individuals either experience a sense of their own historical significance and generate meaning and wisdom, or they fall into existential despair. Tornstam (2005) further elaborated on Erikson's theory, proposing a ninth stage occurring at age 80 and beyond termed *gerotranscendence*. During this stage individuals shift into a *metaprospective* state in a quest to answer existential questions, develop a sense of "cosmic connection" or spirituality, and find a general sense of well-being. Overall, an understanding of how developmental stages can influence an older individual's behavior, choices, and goals across residential settings helps geropsychologists engage in ethical practice that respects both Principle A (Beneficence and Nonmaleficence) and Principle E (Respect for People's Rights and Dignity).

In Elder's (1985, 1998) life course theory, the *life course* is defined as a sequence of socially defined events and roles that the individual enacts over time (Giele & Elder, 1998). This perspective emphasizes the ways in which an individual's socioeconomic culture, the historical period in which he or she lives, and his or her unique internal and interpersonal context influence development. The theory is based on the interaction of four factors: (a) historical time and place, (b) timing in lives, (c) interdependent or linked lives, and (d) human agency. The principle of historical time and place acknowledges the cultural influences of cohort on development and perspective taking. For example, individuals who were born in the 1920s and were in their 70s at the time of the terrorist attacks on the World Trade Center and Pentagon (September 11, 2001) likely experienced and interpreted the events quite differently than individuals who were born in the 1950s and were middle-aged at the time. The second principle, timing in lives, describes the influence of the social clock (Neugarten, 1972); specifically, losing a spouse or sibling is experienced as "off time" if the bereaved individual is a 20- or 30-year-old rather than a 70- or 80-year-old. The third principle of interdependent or linked lives acknowledges the influence of environmental context or the situational imperative, meaning that survival or success depends upon the individual's ability to adapt to the needs of the social and environmental situation at hand. The principle of human agency acknowledges the freedom of individuals to make autonomous choices, consistent with Principle E (Respect for People's Rights and Dignity) in the *Ethical Principles of Psychologists and Code of Conduct* (American Psychological Association, 2010; hereinafter, Ethics Code). Practicing geropsychologists (including those engaged primarily in research) benefit from knowledge of Elder's theory by enhancing communication with the older client through an understanding of cohort, timing, and environmental issues as they pertain to the older individual's choices and needs.

Several theories highlight motivational shifts associated with adult development. Baltes and Baltes's (1990) metamodel *selective optimization with compensation* acknowledges the lifelong process of gains and losses and highlights *selection* as a strategy to maximize emotional outcomes. Older adults evaluate their personal and environmental resources as they relate to individual goals and allocate resources toward goals deemed most important and achievable. *Optimization* refers to the means by which older individuals acquire and refine resources and new skills to pursue and achieve identified goals. *Compensation* refers to functional responses to the loss of goal-relevant means (Boerner & Jopp, 2007) by activating alternative internal and external resources. For example, an older adult with hearing impairment who loves to sing and read may choose to spend more time reading than participating in a choir.

Socioemotional selectivity theory (Carstensen, Isaacowitz, & Charles, 1999) grew out of the selective optimization with compensation metamodel. This well-validated and frequently cited theory posits that as an individual's time perspective becomes more limited rather than open-ended (e.g., time to death becomes shorter and more salient), older adults shift their motivation and behavior to prioritize emotion regulation rather than knowledge acquisition. This shift manifests in a number of ways, such as (a) the pruning of social support networks, (b) positive memory distortion for past choices and autobiographical information, and (c) greater recall of newly presented positively valenced information in comparison with younger adults (Mather & Carstensen, 2005).

Charles (2010) proposed an extended theory, the strength and vulnerability integration model, to describe how emotion regulation changes in older adulthood. In contrast with prior theories, this model acknowledges age-related vulnerabilities in modulating high and sustained physiological arousal. This reduced physiological flexibility may result in delayed recovery from stressful events, moderating the general tendency toward positivity. The application of this set of theories to the ethical practice of geropsychology calls attention to the dialectic between Principle A (Beneficence and Nonmaleficence) and Principle E (Respect for People's Rights and Dignity). Effective geropsychologists attempt to balance an older adult's vulnerabilities with autonomous choices to maximize emotional well-being.

The last set of theories that can be seen as underlying the ethical practice of geropsychology comprises the motivational theory of lifespan development (Heckhausen, Wrosch, & Schulz, 2010). The original lifespan theory of control (Heckhausen & Schulz, 1995) suggested that individuals engage in primary control when it is possible to change the environment to be in line with one's wishes. In contrast, secondary control processes are used when primary control is not possible; in this instance, individuals change themselves to coincide with environmental limitations. Together these two processes optimize an individual's sense of mastery. As an individual ages and loses capacity to respond fully to every environmental challenge, secondary control processes are engaged more frequently. Empirical research and further refinement of this theory (Heckhausen et al., 2010) suggest that older adults optimize their success experiences by refining their goals in line with individual and environmental changes. This theory differs from selective optimization with compensation (Baltes & Baltes, 1990) in that no control strategy may be labeled as adaptive per se, only to the extent that engagement in such strategies supports functionality. Individuals engage and disengage in pursuit of life-relevant goals in line with developmental and environmental needs. Knowledge of this theory and these control processes may enhance ethical practice by enabling the geropsychologist to assist the individual in balancing autonomy and safety in their life choices (e.g., as described in Principles A and E).

PRIMARY GEROPSYCHOLOGY SUBSPECIALTIES AND WORK SETTINGS

Having acquired foundational competency in theoretical and empirical areas of geropsychology, the geropsychologist engaging in ethical practice is competent in multiple practice activities, including assessment, intervention, and consultation. These functional skills may be expressed in a broad range of specialty areas and practice settings, including traditional office-based private practice, mental health outpatient clinics and inpatient settings, home-based care, hospitals, community-based primary care, long-term care, and palliative care and hospice settings. Geropsychologists may also consult with elder law clinics or private law firms regarding the capacity of older individuals to make autonomous choices and engage in instrumental and basic activities of daily living. Additionally, geropsychology services are increasingly being provided in less traditional settings, such as prisons, and through new methods, such as telehealth technology.

Karel and colleagues (Karel, Emery, Molinari, & the CoPGTP Task Force on the Assessment of Geropsychology Competencies, 2010) developed a self-assessment tool for students and professionals at any stage in their career to evaluate their functional competencies in accordance with the Pikes Peak model (Knight, Karel, Hinrichsen, Qualls, & Duffy, 2009). This tool demonstrates preliminary evidence of validity (Karel, Holley, et al., 2012). Molinari (2012) provided further detailed suggestions for meeting knowledge- and skills-based competencies delineated in the Pikes Peak training model, including tables with benchmark descriptions of content for competence in assessment, intervention, consultation, research, supervision training, and management administration.

In terms of assessment, geropsychologists routinely use psychological and cognitive screening instruments as well as self-report and collateral report of an older adult's emotional and behavioral functioning. Some geropsychologists seek advanced training in neuropsychology, although it should be noted that in 2001, the National Academy of Neuropsychology defined a *neuropsychologist* as a psychologist "with special expertise in the applied science of brain–behavior relationships." Neuropsychologists may use their advanced knowledge in assessment, diagnosis, treatment, and rehabilitation of individuals across the lifespan who have experienced neurological, neurodevelopmental, medical, or psychiatric conditions that affect brain–behavior functioning. Thus, neuropsychologists may focus their practice in gerontology, and appropriately trained geropsychologists may also engage in cognitive assessment. In keeping within Standard 2: Competence, which requires that individuals practice within their boundaries of competence, geropsychologists working with older adults practice more broadly and should not purport to be specialists in neuropsychology or brain–behavior relationships unless they have also received advanced training and supervision in this area.

One noteworthy specialty practice area within geropsychology is long-term care practice. This specialty area spans assessment, intervention, and consultation. Psychologists in Long-Term Care (PLTC; http://pltcweb.org) is a network of psychologists and other professionals dedicated to providing high quality mental health services to older adults across the long-term care continuum, including nursing homes, rehabilitation settings, assisted living facilities, and congregate housing. Services provided by PLTC members include individual, group, and family therapy; emotional, behavioral, and cognitive assessment; patient care planning; research; and facility staff training and consultation.

A growing number of geropsychologists work in primary care or palliative and hospice care settings as part of interdisciplinary teams (Haley, Larson, Kasl-Godley, Neimeyer, & Kwilosz, 2003; Karel, Knight, Duffy, Hinrichsen, & Zeiss, 2010; Nydegger, 2008; Zeiss & Steffen, 1996). Nydegger (2008) surveyed 94 community-based hospice programs, however, and found that only seven used psychologists as service providers, and among those seven programs only 17.43% of mental health services were provided by psychologists. Psychologists are much more prevalent mental health service providers in Veterans Affairs (VA) treatment settings, and these settings are typically models of interprofessional care (Karlin & Karel, 2014).

In all such settings, Principle B (Fidelity and Responsibility) and Principle C (Integrity) take on greater importance. To establish trusting working relationships, geropsychologists clearly differentiate their roles within the health care team and communicate effectively with accuracy, honesty, and truthfulness (Integrity). Geropsychologists also advocate for justice in access to services and participation in clinical trials, partially through an understanding of individual, cultural, and cohort differences (Principle D: Justice).

INTERDISCIPLINARY TEAMS AND GEROPSYCHOLOGY

As experts in human behavior and the influence of individual (including cognitive, emotional, and motivational), cultural, and cohort differences, geropsychologists have the opportunity to serve as integral members of interdisciplinary health care teams (O'Shea Carney, Gum, & Zeiss, 2015). For example, Karlin and Karel (2014) examined the extent to which mental health care practices had been integrated nationally into VA home-based primary care teams. They found that psychologists' time was focused on clients with depression, anxiety, caregiver, or family stress; those coping with illness and disability; and cognitive assessment. Moreover, they found that while approximately 40% of providers' time was spent in direct clinical care, significant time was also devoted to team activities, transportation, and charting. The American Psychological Association's policy on psychologists' roles in integrated health care includes (a) diagnosing and treating behavioral health problems, (b) assessment, (c) early intervention and wellness services, (d) outcomes assessment, and (e) development of empirically based interventions (American Psychological Association Presidential Task Force on Integrated Health Care for an Aging Population, 2008). Recent national policy changes, including the rollout of the Patient Protection and Affordable Care Act of 2010 and the emergence of medical homes as a model of interdisciplinary care, may facilitate increased integration of geropsychologists into previously underrepresented practice settings such as hospice and palliative care. Additionally, referrals from elder law clinics and community-based attorneys are likely to increase as the need for capacity evaluations increases (American Bar Association/American Psychological Association Assessment of Capacity in Older Adults Project Working Group, 2008).

Interdisciplinary care can facilitate ethical practice. Given the common developmental decline of individual autonomy as health worsens, and health service providers' dual sense of beneficent responsibility and investment in promoting the autonomy of patients, geropsychologists must develop competencies related to work in interdisciplinary teams (Molinari, 2012; O'Shea Carney et al., 2015). The salient ethical principles in interdisciplinary teamwork include Principles B (Fidelity and Responsibility) and Principle C (Integrity). Differences may arise within interdisciplinary teams, however, because of diverse ethical priorities across disciplines (e.g., the relative importance of respect for autonomy vs. beneficence), lack of understanding of the roles of specific team members, ineffective communication or use of jargon, and inattention to the development of common goals and interests across disciplines (Engel & Prentice, 2013). Mitchell, Parker, Giles, and Boyle (2014) found that conflict may actually increase in more diverse interdisciplinary teams, but only when multiple team members strongly endorse professional identification over team identification. For example, in an interdisciplinary team within VA Community Living Centers or in community nursing homes consisting of nursing and psychology, robust and (hopefully) productive discussions about the availability of coffee to residents may illustrate divergent commitment to safety (e.g., nursing staff concerns that residents may burn themselves) versus autonomous choice (e.g., residents enjoy the availability of coffee through-out the day, a psychological benefit). Such conflict may decrease as a function of effective communication and open-mindedness. Mitchell and colleagues (2014) found that dysfunctional interdisciplinary team functioning was mini-mized within the context of transformational leadership, reinforcement of shared values and goals, and the development of a shared group identity.

INDIVIDUAL, CULTURAL, AND COHORT DIFFERENCES

Elder's (1985, 1998) life course theory serves as an excellent theoretical underpinning for consideration of individual, cultural, and cohort differences in the ethical practice of geropsychology. Respecting individual differences reflects support for agency and is emphasized in Principle E (Respect for People's Rights and Dignity). Cultural or environmental characteristics (Elder's [1985, 1998] interconnected or linked lives), including access to quality education and health care, directly influence the options available to older individuals, and geropsychologists must be aware of how such characteristics may or may not reflect appropriate availability of services (Principle D: Justice). Finally, cohort differences reflect Elder's (1985, 1998) notions about the influence of historical time and place on health behavior and again pertain to the principle of justice. Health disparities are caused by poverty, poor access to health and mental health care, and educational differences. Other factors often associated with health disparities include cultural and cohort factors that reduce the abil-ity to achieve the best health and mental health outcomes among minority or otherwise underserved groups. These groups may include but are not limited to older adults, people of color, women, those with low education and income, rural-dwelling individuals, and sexual and gender minorities (e.g., lesbian, gay, bisexual, transgender; Centers for Disease Control and Prevention, 2012). Geropsychologists must strive to decrease these disparities through advocacy or pro-bono social justice activities and engagement.

CONCLUSION

The emergence of geropsychology as a subspecialty of clinical psychol-ogy is based on its unique contributions to understanding and serving older adults. Competent practice requires an understanding of the integration of psychology and gerontology, including a solid foundation in developmental theories. Such foundational knowledge may directly influence ethical practice, as noted previously in the discussion of American Psychological Association (2010) ethical principles as they relate to developmental theory. Geropsychologists, having broad-based knowledge and skills, commonly further specialize in their activities, the specific older adult population, or the settings in which services are provided. Work within interdisciplinary teams and consultation with colleagues from other disciplines are typically valuable roles for geropsychologists, facilitating comprehensive care of older adults. Relative to younger adult populations, the practice of geropsychology more likely entails close interaction with the older adult client's family members or other caregivers. Efforts to understand individual, cultural, and cohort differences among older adult clients are essential to the effective practice of geropsychology. This integration of psychology and gerontology underlies the ethical practice of geropsychology.

2

ESTABLISHING AND MAINTAINING COMPETENCE IN GEROPSYCHOLOGY

The quality of a person's life is in direct proportion to their commitment
to excellence, regardless of their chosen field of endeavor.
—Vince Lombardi

Professional competence is the foundation upon which ethical practice in psychology and its specialties, including geropsychology, is built.
Consistent with the ethical principles of beneficence and nonmaleficence
(Principle A; American Psychological Association [APA], 2010), professional competence improves the likelihood that psychological services are
beneficial to older adults and other involved parties and reduces the potential
for harmful outcomes. Education, training, and professional experience are
the building blocks of professional competence. Inadequate education and
training and lack of experience with older adults reduce the likelihood that
elder patients will benefit from the services provided and increase the potential for harmful effects to individuals and to the reputation of geropsychology
from unnecessary or inappropriate services. In geropsychology, perhaps more
than in some psychological specialties, personal life experiences and cohort
issues combine with education, training, and professional experience to contribute to the professional development of the clinician. Personal experiences

http://dx.doi.org/10.1037/0000010-003
Ethical Practice in Geropsychology, by S. S. Bush, R. S. Allen, and V. A. Molinari

interacting with older adult relatives or members of the elder community can give clinicians firsthand knowledge of both the positive aspects and the challenges of aging, which has the potential to enrich clinical experiences with older adult patients. (Such experiences, however, do not substitute for formal education and training.) As mentioned in Chapter 1, foundational knowledge of developmental theories that consider the impact of cohort or historical time and place (e.g., Elder's [1985, 1998] life course theory) contributes strongly to geropsychologists' ethical practice.

The *Ethical Principles of Psychologists and Code of Conduct* (APA, 2010) states,

> Where scientific or professional knowledge in the discipline of psychology establishes that an understanding of factors associated with age . . . is essential for effective implementation of their services or research, psychologists have or obtain the training, experience, consultation or supervision necessary to ensure the competence of their services, or they make appropriate referrals, except as provided in Standard 2.02, Providing Services in Emergencies.

When planning to begin working with new populations, psychologists have an ethical obligation to "undertake relevant education, training, supervised experience, consultation or study" (Standard 2.01c).

The U.S. population is aging, the new cohort of older adults is more receptive to mental health services, service settings for older adults are increasing, and market forces are changing, all of which results in considerable need for psychologists who are proficient in the provision of clinical services to older adults (APA, 2014c; Vincent & Velkoff, 2010). However, widespread preparation by the profession to meet the psychological needs of older adults is lacking. Graduate training in professional psychology continues to be under pressure to respond to the growing number of older adults and their mental health needs (e.g., Allen, Crowther, & Molinari, 2013; Hinrichsen, Zeiss, Karel, & Molinari, 2010; Karel, Gatz, & Smyer, 2012; Qualls, Scogin, Zweig, & Whitbourne, 2010). A survey of practicing psychologists determined that fewer than 30% had any graduate coursework in geropsychology, fewer than 20% had any supervised practicum or internship experience with this population, and more than 50% of the respondents indicated that additional training was needed (Qualls, Segal, Norman, Niederehe, & Gallagher-Thompson, 2002). Packard (2007) found that while 70% of psychologists have older adult patients, only 3% have had formal geropsychology training. Although gains in this area have likely been made in the past decade, the shortage of clinicians who are qualified to work with older adults remains (Clay, 2006; Rosen, 2005). Indeed, although graduates of programs that focus on work with older adults believe their clinical and research training was strong, they rated training in teaching and supervision less highly (Carpenter, Sakai, Karel, Molinari, & Moye, 2016; Karel, Sakai, Molinari, Moye, & Carpenter, 2016). Teaching of geropsychology and supervising student work with older adults is obviously necessary to bridge the increasing demand for services in the absence of an adequate supply of competent practitioners. The profession has a responsibility to strive to remedy this demand–supply chasm, and individual psychologists working with older adults have an ethical obligation to establish and maintain the knowledge base and skills needed to promote the care and wellbeing of their patients.

EDUCATION AND TRAINING IN GEROPSYCHOLOGY

Competent professional and ethical practice in geropsychology does not consistently happen by chance. Preparation is the key to establishing professional competence in geropsychology and reflects the proactive commitment to ethical practice that is advanced by positive ethics. Although there can be multiple paths to competent practice with older adults, the optimal path is structured, comprehensive, and supervised, rather than informal or piecemeal. To meet the APA Commission on Accreditation's aspirational goal of providing truly broad and general training, issues of adult development and aging and exposure to clinical experiences with aging adults need to be incorporated into all existing doctoral training programs.

Formal education in geropsychology allows students to obtain the knowledge and expertise they need for clinical practice, research, and other professional activities provided to, or on behalf of, older adults. Such education, integrating clinical psychology and gerontology, may occur at the undergraduate or predoctoral level but usually begins during doctoral education (Allen, Crowther, & Molinari, 2013). Often, general courses on adult development and aging are offered, with more specific topics covered in subsequent courses. Training is the process through which students or others new to the specialty obtain the experience and develop the skills to apply the didactic knowledge needed for the competent practice of geropsychology. Such training often begins with practicum/externship experiences, is included in internships, and becomes the sole focus at the postdoctoral residency level.

The APA (2014c) *Guidelines for Psychological Practice With Older Adults*, which outlines areas of competence for the practice of geropsychology, is organized and provides recommendations around six themes: (a) competence and attitudes; (b) general knowledge about adult development, aging, and older adults; (c) clinical issues; (d) assessment; (e) intervention, consultation, and other service provision; and (f) professional issues and education. In addition to these guidelines, the Pikes Peak training model (Knight, Karel, Hinrichsen, Qualls, & Duffy, 2009) provides detailed guidance for acquiring the recommended competencies. The comprehensive competencies described in the Pikes Peak model emphasize self-evaluation and supervisee ratings in core knowledge and skill areas, reflecting diversity in clinical activities, care settings, and demographic and sociocultural factors (Council of Professional Geropsychology Training Programs, 2013; Molinari, 2012). Typically, the attainment of professional competence in geropsychology is a process that spans multiple programs at different levels of education and training, including graduate education, internship, postdoctoral residency, and postlicensure education and training.

EDUCATION AND TRAINING IN ETHICS

Professional competence in geropsychology is not limited to developing knowledge and skills for working with older adults. Clinicians must also establish and maintain ethical competence—that is, education and training in the ethical and legal aspects of practice, including ethical decision making, are critical for establishing professional competence. Such preparation can include formal coursework, didactic seminars, journal clubs, case conferences, and individual supervision. Because ethics underlie all professional behavior, there should never be a time when a supervisee reports there are "no ethical issues" to discuss.

SUPERVISION

The development of competent clinical skills largely depends on the quality of the supervision received by trainees. Clinical supervision has been described as a central component of training in psychology (Romans, Boswell, Carlozzi, & Ferguson, 1995) and as "the critical teaching method" (Holloway, 1992, p. 177; see also Falender & Shafranske, 2007). In professional health-service psychology, which includes geropsychology, supervision is the most frequently used method for teaching a variety of skills, including assessment, report writing, differential diagnosis, and treatment (Falender & Shafranske, 2004). Additionally, the provision of supervision to trainees, junior colleagues, and other professionals is a job requirement for many psychologists (Sutter, McPherson, & Geeseman, 2002) and is often assigned prematurely (Barnett, Erickson Cornish, Goodyear, & Lichtenberg, 2007).

Formal development of foundational and functional supervisory competencies has traditionally been absent from psychology education and training programs. Peake, Nussbaum, and Tindell (2002) reported that less than 20% of supervisors in clinical psychology had received any formal training in supervision. Rather, it was widely assumed that good clinicians would make good supervisors, that patient care and supervisory skills are so closely related that they transfer without the need for additional training. This traditional assumption has been recognized in recent years as being false, resulting in more emphasis being placed on training clinicians to be supervisors. In 2006, APA published guidelines stating that clinical supervision is to be considered a specific professional competency (APA, 2014b), and psychology as a profession has increased its focus on competencies, training standards, site reviews, and postdoctoral subspecialties (France et al., 2008). Therefore, consistent with ethical requirements (Standard 2.01, Boundaries of Competence), effective supervisors must be competent in supervision as well as in the professional activities they are supervising.

Effective supervisors share the following qualities: (a) interest in training; (b) availability; (c) flexibility; (d) respectfulness of trainees; (e) supportiveness, rather than being overly critical or punitive; (f) ability to cultivate the supervisory relationship into one that is trusting, collaborative, and honest; (g) ability to cultivate an atmosphere of intellectual, clinical, and professional curiosity; and (h) an emotional investment in the trainee's professional development (Stucky, Bush, & Donders, 2010; see also Chapter 7, this volume, for supervision and mentorship in teaching and research). An evaluation process that includes 360-degree feedback (i.e., self-evaluation and direct feedback from trainees, colleagues, and supervisors) can help supervisors achieve and maintain the qualities of an effective supervisor. When inviting feedback, supervisors are open to, and accepting of, negative feedback and use the information for professional growth or discussion of the trainee's or others' expectations. Effective supervisors recognize that the power differential between supervisor and supervisee may prevent some trainees from initiating discussion of concerns or dissatisfaction, which makes active elicitation of feedback from trainees a particularly important supervisor function.

Goals of Supervision

The primary purpose of supervision in geropsychology is to develop competent geropsychologists, with the overarching goal of protecting older adult patients, the public, and the profession. This goal is achieved by facilitating the development of (a) geropsychological knowledge and skills, (b) critical thinking and decision making, (c) effective clinical care, (d) investment in career-long learning, (e) meaningful patient outcomes, and (f) essential attitudes for ethical practice (e.g., respect for others, honesty, integrity). To achieve these interrelated goals, supervisors foster a close mentoring relationship that promotes a transformative process on multiple levels, allowing trainees to advance professional and technical competence while establishing a professional identity.

Supervisors have a considerable effect, either positive or negative, on trainee professional self-esteem, competence, identity, values, and biases. Effective supervisors model professional behavior, introduce systems level thinking, provide advanced training in the application of various skills in multiple patient and nonpatient care venues, and allow for the mutual consideration of complex ethical and diversity issues, barriers to the efficient and appropriate delivery of patient care, educational initiatives, and professional obligations (Stucky et al., 2010). Given the breadth and complexity of supervision, it is understandable that trainees and supervisors can experience dissatisfaction if the purpose, structure, and expectations for supervision are not clearly established and followed.

Models of Supervision

The value of health-service psychology specialties, including geropsychology, is based on the provision of quality supervision to its trainees and is shaped by their selection of trainees, education and training standards, expected competencies, and the structure of their training programs (Patterson & Hanson, 1995; Stiers & Stucky, 2008). Quality training programs are typically guided by a model that facilitates the conceptualization and structuring of supervision. Many models of supervision are available in professional psychology (Falender & Shafranske, 2004; Kaufman & Kaufman, 2006). Three common general approaches to supervision focus on (a) administrative issues, (b) clinical issues, and (c) supervisee psychotherapy. It has been recommended that supervisors utilize a competency-based, metatheoretical approach, which involves working within any theoretical or practice modality; is science-informed, formalized, and objective; and systematically considers the growth of specific competencies in the development of overall professional competence (APA, 2015).

To the extent possible, supervisory competencies correspond to foundational and functional competencies in professional psychology in general (Rodolfa et al., 2005) and in geropsychology more specifically. Psychology supervisors need the following foundational competencies: (a) reflective practice (self-assessment), (b) scientific knowledge and methods, (c) relationships, (d) individual and cultural diversity, (e) ethical and legal standards and policy issues, and (f) interdisciplinary systems. Functional competencies for psychology supervisors include (a) assessment-diagnosis-case conceptualization, (b) intervention, (c) consultation, (d) research evaluation, (e) supervision training, and (f) management and administration (Fouad et al., 2009; Rodolfa et al., 2005). Supervisors also model respectful and appropriate professional behavior. Ethical supervisors provide supervision of professional activities in which they possess specific training or competence, delegating to colleagues supervision of activities for which their competence is lacking.

Supervision, particularly with postdoctoral fellows, should include business aspects of geropsychology practice. Teaching residents about billing and reimbursement; institutional governance structure, priorities, dynamics, and politics; and risk management can enhance the preparation of trainees for conducting ethical clinical practice. Training programs are "designed to provide the appropriate knowledge and proper experiences, and to meet the requirements for licensure, certification or other goals for which claims are made by the program" (Standard 7.01, Design of Education and Training Programs). In terms of evaluating supervisee performance, competent supervisors "establish a timely and specific process for providing feedback to students and supervisees. Information regarding the process is provided to the student at the beginning of supervision" (Standard 7.06, Assessing Student and Supervisee Performance). Supervisors understand the differences between formative evaluation (i.e., periodic evaluation and feedback during the process of training) and summative evaluation (i.e., meeting specific program exit criteria; Stucky et al., 2010).

Barriers to Training in Supervision

Establishing competence in supervision is not always a seamless process. The hierarchical medical model whereby faculty/staff train and supervise senior trainees who in turn train and supervise more junior trainees is not always possible; in some settings senior trainees may have limited access to junior trainees for supervisory opportunities. Given the limited number of experts in geropsychology, faculty and staff with extensive experience providing services to older adults and their families may not be available. As mentioned previously, a recent survey found that even students who have completed geropsychology graduate or postdoctoral programs report that training in supervision is weak relative to training in clinical work (Karel et al., 2016). The most common barriers to training in supervision include counterproductive personality dynamics, contrasting supervisory styles, disagreements among supervisory faculty, unclear evaluation procedures, and vague goals (Stucky et al., 2010).

Responsibility and Legal Liability

According to state licensing laws, supervisors are legally liable for negligence if they do not supervise adequately (direct liability) and for the actions of supervisees, even if the supervisor performed competently as a supervisor (vicarious liability; Falender & Shafranske, 2013; Saccuzzo, 2015). Well-meaning but unprepared psychologists who lack foundational and functional competence in geropsychology may not recognize the demands or complexities of supervision until they have had negative supervisory experiences or outcomes. A proactive approach to supervisory competence helps to promote positive supervisory experiences for supervisors, trainees, and the patients and systems they serve. One means of obtaining such supervision by "bona fide professional geropsychologists" (Knight et al., 2009, p. 210) may be web-based consultation services.

An important function of supervisors in the promotion of patient care and protection of the public is serving as gatekeepers who can dissuade geropsychology trainees from practice if they are not in the right specialty or modify trainees' educational programs and supervision to maximize their potential to work through or resolve glaring weaknesses. To say that providing unfavorable feedback to a trainee can be disheartening for the trainee and difficult for the supervisor is an understatement. However, critical feedback provided in a supportive, educational manner can protect trainees from more severe consequences for incompetent practice later in a career, protect future patients, and protect the integrity of the training program and the reputation of geropsychology as a field of practice. Such actions demonstrate to trainees the importance of ethical practice as a clinician and supervisor. "Valuing and modeling ethical behavior and adherence to relevant legal and regulatory parameters in supervision is essential to upholding the highest duty of the supervisor, protecting the public" (APA, 2015, p. 41).

REFLECTIVE PRACTICE

Although negative experiences provide a natural point for reflecting on the nature and quality of one's practices, self-assessment is a process best performed at regular intervals, even when supervisory experiences by all accounts have been successful. Completion of the *Pikes Peak Geropsychology Knowledge and Assessment Tool* (Council of Professional Geropsychology Training Programs, 2013) as part of the supervisory process with trainees affords supervisors an excellent opportunity to reflect on their own knowledge and skills at least once a year. The tenets of the Pike's Peak training model have been validated (Wharton, Shah, Scogin, & Allen, 2013), and the Pikes Peak Geropsychology Knowledge and Assessment Tool (Karel, Emery, Molinari, & the CoPGTP Task Force on the Assessment of Geropsychology Competencies, 2010) shows preliminary evidence of validity (Karel, Holley, et al., 2012). As previously described, an evaluation process that includes 360-degree feedback also provides supervisors an opportunity to review their own strengths and weaknesses and to develop a plan to continue their professional development.

Countertransference

Assessing and addressing countertransference can be an important part of developing appropriate clinical skills with older adults. Most people have ideas about what it means to age, about successful aging, and about aspects of older adulthood that may be considered disappointing, dissatisfying, or disgusting, and psychologists are no exception. Such ageist beliefs and the emotions that accompany the beliefs have the potential to influence clinical judgments, choices, and actions. The influences may be positive, facilitating rapport and promoting patient care, or negative, resulting in the substitution of clinician values for patient values and the provision or denial of services in a manner that is inconsistent with the patient's wishes or needs. Being aware of ageist beliefs fueling countertransference and its potential impact on professional services allows geropsychologists to make more informed decisions and facilitates appropriate care. Maintaining awareness of ageist beliefs and striving to counter such beliefs help maximize the rights and well-being of older adults by preventing unfair discrimination against them (Standard 3.01, Unfair Discrimination).

Professionalism

Consistent with countertransference, sometimes working with older adults leads clinicians to think of patients like older adult relatives, with a resulting temptation to become less formal in their manner of interaction and even to be less prone to use confrontation when appropriate (Knight, 2004). Informality may be evident by using a less formal method of addressing the patient, such as "poppa." Such "elderspeak" (Kemper & Harden, 1999) may also be evident in the adoption of a more chatty than psychotherapeutic interaction. Such informality may be culturally or clinically appropriate in a given case; however, competent geropsychologists weigh the potential advantages and disadvantages of various ways of interacting with patients before doing so and make such decisions on the basis of the patient's best interests and, when possible, empirical evidence.

BOARD CERTIFICATION

Attainment of board certification in geropsychology through the American Board of Professional Psychology provides the clearest evidence of professional competence in geropsychology. Although board certification in a specialty does not imply expertise in all facets of the specialty (e.g., all of the various clinical settings, assessment and treatment methods, and unique patient subpopulations), it does reflect possession of core foundational and functional competencies that are valued by the specialty overall (Allen, Crowther, & Molinari, 2013). Completion of this formal, reasonably rigorous peer review process helps protect consumers from substandard services by providing a recognizable sign of professional competence in the specialty. Although a clinician's lack of board certification in geropsychology does not necessarily imply a lack of knowledge and skills in this specialty, it is difficult for employers or consumers to distinguish those who are qualified from those who are not when clinicians do not have the credential. As consumers continue to become more sophisticated about professional credentials, and as board certification in psychology continues to grow, board certification may one day become expected by older adult patients and their representatives (as well as employers of geropsychologists), as it is in medicine.

MAINTAINING COMPETENCE

Professional competence is not all-encompassing or permanent. Even if the science of gerontology and geropsychology was not advancing at an explosive rate, there would be enough for practitioners at all career stages to learn and improve upon to fill conference programming for many years. As it is, because of the comprehensive knowledge and skill set required of geropsychologists and rapid advances in science and professional literature, the ethical mandate to maintain competence (Standard 2.03, Maintaining Competence) has essentially become an endeavor that is integrated into daily practice. There are numerous resources to which clinicians can turn to find answers to, and expand understanding of, clinical challenges that emerge in routine practice. Journals, essential textbooks, position statements from professional organizations, local grand rounds, reputable websites, formal continuing education courses, and informal exchanges with colleagues are examples of resources that can promote professional competence, but such resources are only of value when clinicians have a personal commitment to maintaining and advancing professional competence. It has been recommended that "there be a culture shift toward a high value on assessing competence across the professional life span" (Kaslow et al., 2007, p. 448). In addition to maintaining competence in geropsychology, continuing education in professional ethics as applied to work with older adults can be particularly valuable and should be pursued. Steady monitoring and self-evaluation using the Pikes Peak Competencies Assessment Tool (Karel, Emery, et al., 2010) can be invaluable in the clinician's endeavor to maintain competence.

GEROPSYCHOLOGICAL SERVICES BY NONGEROPSYCHOLOGISTS

Psychologists who have not been educated and trained in geropsychology may ethically assess and treat older adults if (a) they are in an underserved location and a more qualified psychologist is unavailable, provided steps are taken to establish their competence (Standard 2.01d, Boundaries of Competence); or (b) they are in an emergency (Standard 2.02, Providing Services in Emergencies). However, psychologists who intend to provide services to older adults on a more consistent basis need to undertake a more systematic effort to ensure their competence. Efforts are currently underway to define the behavioral descriptors of basic foundational competencies so that continuing education programs can reflect their core content. As Standard 2.01c (Boundaries of Competence) states, "Psychologists planning to provide services, teach or conduct research involving populations, areas, techniques, or technologies new to them undertake relevant education, training, supervised experience, consultation or study." Typically, some combination of these education and training activities is needed.

CONCLUSION

The ethical practice of geropsychology requires professional competence in order for clinicians to provide services that benefit rather than harm older adults (Principle A: Beneficence and Nonmaleficence). Establishing professional competence in geropsychology may begin with undergraduate and graduate education and certainly continues with predoctoral or postdoctoral supervised training (Allen, Crowther, & Molinari, 2013). The Pikes Peak Geropsychology Knowledge and Assessment Tool details the foundational and functional competencies required of geropsychologists (Karel, Knight, Duffy, Hinrichsen, & Zeiss, 2010). Supervision itself is also a professional competency that is developed in the same manner as other professional skills. Successful completion of a formal peer review examination process (i.e., board certification in geropsychology) provides the clearest evidence of professional competence in geropsychology and serves as an indicator to the public and other professionals that the professional is qualified to provide clinical services to older adults. Maintaining professional competence requires a proactive, personal investment in staying abreast of emerging scientific and professional literature. Particularly invested clinicians may wish to not simply maintain competence but also to expand areas of knowledge and improve or expand skill sets. Given the advancing age of the U.S. population, the receptivity of the new cohort of older adults to mental health services, and changing service settings and market forces, the need for competent geropsychologists has never been greater.

3

ETHICAL ISSUES AND DECISION MAKING IN GEROPSYCHOLOGY

We do not act rightly because we have virtue or excellence, but we rather have those because we have acted rightly.

—Aristotle

The term *ethical issues* is sometimes used interchangeably with *ethical dilemmas*; however, they are not the same. There are ethical issues in all clinical activities. General bioethical principles, represented in the General Principles section of the American Psychological Association's (APA; 2010) *Ethical Principles of Psychologists and Code of Conduct* (hereinafter, Ethics Code), underlie and guide clinical and other professional services in psychology. Ethical Standards and other professional guidelines provide additional direction for psychologists, including those working with older adults; the standards are enforceable and the guidelines are considered aspirational. For example, fundamental activities such as obtaining informed consent (or assent) from patients involve ethical principles (i.e., respect for patient autonomy) are represented by specific ethical standards in the Ethics Code (Standards 3.10, 8.02, 8.03, 8.05, 9.03, and 10.01), and are thus ethical issues. In most instances, such ethical issues are managed in a routine manner and no challenges arise. Psychologists, however, should strive to incorporate conscious consideration

http://dx.doi.org/10.1037/0000010-004
Ethical Practice in Geropsychology, by S. S. Bush, R. S. Allen, and V. A. Molinari

of ethics into daily practice. Depending on one's practice setting and specific patient population, some ethical issues may be more prevalent than others.

Ethical issues are most likely to become challenges when (a) they pit ethical, legal, or organizational requirements against one another; (b) the Ethics Code or laws are silent on the issue, such as with relatively new areas of practice; or (c) they require the professional to rely on judgment. Ethically complex situations and inconsistencies among sources of authority can make optimal decisions difficult to discern. Competing ethical principles are common sources of dilemmas for clinicians (Beauchamp & Childress, 2013). For example, respect for patient autonomy may conflict with the principle of beneficence when a patient who is cognitively intact does not consent to a procedure that is considered by clinicians to be essential for the patient's well-being. This conflict between respect for patient autonomy and beneficence reflects an ethical dilemma and a clinical challenge for care providers. This chapter reviews common ethical issues and dilemmas in psychological practice with older adults and offers a decision-making model for addressing the issues and resolving the dilemmas.

COMMON ETHICAL ISSUES AND CHALLENGES

The ethical principles and standards that guide clinicians and govern the practice of clinical psychology with younger populations also apply to and inform psychologists working with older adults. However, geropsychologists are likely to find some ethical issues to be of more immediate relevance or more commonly the source of dilemmas than issues that are more relevant to younger adult populations.

Bush (2012) reviewed the literature and drew from personal experience to propose eight aspects of practice with older adults that are of primary ethical importance: (a) professional competence; (b) human relations (including family members, peers, caregivers, and health care institutions), confidentiality, and informed consent; (c) assessment; (d) treatment; (e) special populations; (f) health promotion; (g) social considerations, and (h) record keeping. These ethical issues can become ethical challenges and dilemmas and are most likely to do so for clinicians who have given little consideration to ethical issues and ways to avoid ethical challenges.

Similarly, Karel (2011) described ethical issues commonly encountered in geropsychology in the context of assessment, intervention, consultation, and research. Issues identified as particularly salient include informed consent (assent, proxy consent), privacy and confidentiality, reliability and validity of tests with older adults, appropriate coding and billing, advocacy and access to needed services, and services delivered to or through organizations (conflicts of interest, reimbursement). Karel also covered decision-making capacity. From the perspective of bioethical principles, Karel noted that, typically, respect for patient autonomy and beneficence are integrated to help guide a plan of care.

Having considered these prior resources, and with an understanding that all of the ethical issues mentioned are of great importance in geropsychology, we focus in this section on four issues that are likely to affect the ethical psychological care of older adults: (a) professional competence, (b) the need to balance the principles of respect for patient autonomy and beneficence within the context of familial and professional support systems, (c) limitations with the evidence base for assessment and treatment, and (d) work with interprofessional teams.

Professional Competence

Competence in geropsychology consists of three overarching components: competence in professional psychology, competence in gerontology, and competence in integrating professional psychology and gerontology. As described in Chapter 2, having appropriate education, training, and experience prepares psychologists to understand these scientific and professional knowledge bases, which underlie psychological services for older adults (Standards 2.01, Boundaries of Competence, and 2.04, Bases for Scientific and Professional Judgments; Knight, Karel, Hinrichsen, Qualls, & Duffy, 2009). The ability to identify and understand ethical and legal aspects of practice and to prevent or address ethical dilemmas is also a component of professional competence. Consistent ethical practice of geropsychology does not happen by chance. Without adequate preparation and maintenance of competence, the potential is great for ineffective or harmful services for patients and damage to the reputation of the profession and the career of the individual practitioner.

Need to Balance Respect for Patient Autonomy With Beneficence

A panel of geropsychologists experienced with ethical issues agreed that balancing the principles of respect for patient autonomy with promotion or protection of patient welfare (i.e., beneficence) is the single greatest ethical challenge facing geropsychologists (Bush, Allen, Heck, & Moye, 2015). Clinicians working with older adults often experience a tension between their desire to support the rights of patients to make the decisions that govern their lives and their investment in promoting patient welfare when patients' decisions appear to be inconsistent with their welfare. This issue becomes even more complicated when patients' decision-making capacity is in question. In this instance, knowledge of the individual's long-term values guiding his or her behaviors across the lifespan is essential.

Personal values drive decisions about how people live their lives, including their later years. Who we want to share our lives with, how we want to spend our time and resources, what types of medical care we accept or reject, and the settings in which we live (or die) are the types of decisions that competent adults expect and have a right to make, often with input from trusted others. For example, some adults believe that quality of life is more important than duration of life and therefore reject life-prolonging procedures that have a high risk of leaving them too compromised to live life as fully as they are used to. Other adults believe that every day is precious and will do whatever they can to have one more minute of life, even with significant limitations. Geropsychologists respect the values and preferences of competent adults, including when those values and preferences are represented by an advance directive or surrogate decision maker. Geropsychologists strive to promote the well-being and care of their older adult patients but not at the expense of the patients' wishes or values. Geropsychologists consider the role that their own values play in their professional activities and decisions but take care not to substitute their own values for those of their patients. The Pikes Peak Competencies Assessment Tool (Karel, Emery, Molinari, & the CoPGTP Task Force on the Assessment of Geropsychology Competencies, 2010; Karel, Molinari, Emery-Tiburcio, & Knight, 2015) assists geropsychologists in performing regular self-evaluations to determine how their personal values may be influencing their ethical practice.

Striving to balance respect for autonomy with beneficence in the context of complex clinical and ethical situations is often a process that relies on the geropsychologist's communication and therapy skills. When the competent older adult patient's wishes appear to conflict with what family members or treatment team members believe is in the patient's best interests, the geropsychologist is often well-positioned to help all parties work toward a solution. Therapy sessions with the patient can help explore and clarify values, consider options in the context of such values, reflect on how various decisions affect those involved in the patient's life, and consider the importance of others' feelings and wishes in the overall decision-making process. Couples or family therapy sessions can contribute to collaborative decision making; however, geropsychologists are aware that strong personalities or family dynamics may sway patients away from their personal values toward decisions that they would otherwise not make.

Geropsychologists can also facilitate communication between the patient, family, and care providers, clarifying for care providers the patient's perspective and why a medically unpopular decision is preferred by the patient and is consistent with the patient's longstanding perspective on life. Consider a situation in which a surgeon instructs the geropsychologist to convince the patient to accept life-saving surgery. The geropsychologist recognizes that the surgeon's belief that he alone knows what is best for the patient is an archaic, paternalistic approach to medicine and that strong interdisciplinary communication skills will be needed to promote understanding in this case. After discussion with all parties, it may be that the geropsychologist needs to explain to the surgeon that the patient's decision to "let nature take its course" is entirely consistent with the value system of (a) the patient and his family, (b) the culture in which they live, and (c) the religion in which they believe, and it is therefore the right decision for the patient. As Karel (2011) stated, "Most often, the principles of autonomy and beneficence coincide to help guide a plan of care; usually patients and health care providers agree, after education and discussion, about the best course of action for the patient" (p. 118).

Limitations With the Evidence Base for Assessment, Treatment, and Health Promotion

Lifespan developmental differences, sensory and motor deficits, increased medical problems and use of medications, and cohort social differences are among the issues that distinguish psychological services provided to older adults from those of younger populations. Considerable advancements have been made in recent years in the development of assessment measures, normative data, treatment approaches, and health promotion options specifically for older adults. Traditionally, however, the evidence bases for such services have lagged behind the evidence bases for younger adult populations or have been extensions of existing models or data sets applied or extended upward in age range rather than being originally conceptualized and developed for use with older adults. Ethical geropsychologists are selective in the use of assessment and treatment methods, understand the advantages and risks of relying on methods developed for younger populations or later-born cohorts, seek empirical evidence to support choice of methods, and are able to describe limitations in services provided based on the methods selected. These issues are covered in more detail in Chapters 4 and 5 in this book.

Work With Interprofessional Teams

Part of the richness and benefit of evaluating and treating older adults is that in many clinical contexts, there is close collaboration with interdisciplinary colleagues. Geropsychologists gain much from the information and perspectives obtained from other professionals and contribute much to the treatment team's understanding of the cognitive, emotional, and behavioral understanding and treatment of older adult patients. Older adults benefit from the exchange and integration of specialized information among their clinical team members. Geropsychologists are also well-positioned, through an understanding of interpersonal and team dynamics that is developed during training and subsequent experience, to facilitate communication among team members and maximize collaboration. Such skills can be extremely helpful to teams as they grapple with challenging clinical situations, personalities, and behaviors.

Conceptualizing and providing care through an interprofessional team perspective is not limited to settings in which formal teams are inherently present. Geropsychologists in independent practice also, with appropriate consent, enhance clinical services by communicating and collaborating with other professionals in the community who provide clinical services to their older adult patients. Like geropsychologists, other professionals in the community tend to understand the value of interprofessional collaboration and are open to, or initiate, contact with geropsychologists. Whether part of a formal interprofessional team or collaborating with other interprofessional colleagues in a private practice context, geropsychologists understand the value of having the older adult patients and their involved family members or other care providers be part of the team whenever possible, and they strive to ensure that other team members maintain that same inclusive perspective.

With the benefits of interprofessional collaboration come ethical challenges. Common challenges include (a) maintaining the balance between sharing patient information and maintaining privacy and confidentiality, (b) cooperating with team members who maintain strict paternalistic or authoritarian stances toward patients and other team members, and (c) maintaining appropriate limits on the roles of psychology when asked to move beyond one's scope of practice or the apparent best interests of a given patient. Frequent, open communication with interprofessional colleagues is typically the preferred approach to limiting and addressing such challenges. Promoting such communication proactively such as through grand rounds or other team educational activities can help avoid some ethical challenges and ease the communication and resolution process that should occur when ethical challenges arise.

ETHICAL AWARENESS IN GEROPSYCHOLOGY

Good clinical practice and sound ethical practice are fundamentally intertwined. Ethical and legal issues underlie all clinical activities, and psychologists who think in those terms on a consistent basis are well-positioned to maximize understanding and promote the well-being of older adults. Whereas all psychology graduate programs require at least one course on psychological ethics, very few, if any, offer courses specific to ethical and legal issues in geropsychology. The development of foundational and functional competencies in geropsychology provides the core of the skill set needed to serve older adults; but the ethical and legal requirements and guidelines provide the road map for applying the skill set in a manner that advances the interests and well-being of older adult clients and minimizes the potential for harmful outcomes, in an atmosphere of integrity and fairness. To meet the APA Committee on Accreditation's goal of broad and general training for all psychologists (APA, 2006), formal education and training in geropsychology ethics and laws is needed in all training programs as well as through continuing education and independent studies throughout the careers of current practitioners (Allen, Crowther, & Molinari, 2013).

AN ETHICAL DECISION-MAKING MODEL IN GEROPSYCHOLOGY

Ethical decision making, like clinical decision making, tends to be most effective when it follows a structured, logical process and is supported by evidence. Psychology scholars have described the potential value of using a systematic approach to ethical decision making (see Knapp & VandeCreek, 2003, for a review). Decision-making models allow clinicians to determine a preferred course of action when faced with competing ethical principles or conflicting directives by clarifying the issues and considering and weighing the relative importance of pertinent information. Such models provide clinicians an outline of important points to consider and a method of examining resources so that sound ethical decisions can be made.

From a pragmatic ethical perspective, what geropsychologists want to know is, "What should I do?" That primary question is answered in what is typically the final or nearly final step in the ethical decision-making process. It is the steps leading up to that answer that position the geropsychologist to make a good decision that is consistent with ethical conduct (see Exhibit 3.1).

EXHIBIT 3.1
Ethical Decision-Making Questions

1. What is the ethical issue?
2. Who are the stakeholders, and what are my obligations to them?
3. What references can help me decide?
4. How might my values and beliefs affect my decisions?
5. What are my options?
6. Which should I do?
7. How did it work out, and is anything else needed?

From their review of several ethical decision-making models, Knapp and VandeCreek (2003) identified five steps that these models had in common: (a) identification of the problem, (b) development of alternatives, (c) evaluation of alternatives, (d) implementation of the best option, and (e) evaluation of the results. Knapp and VandeCreek also noted that the models reviewed did not adequately consider emotional and situational factors or the possible need for an immediate response. Reflecting an understanding of a systematic, step-by-step approach to ethical decision making, the Canadian Psychological Association (2000) included a 10-step ethical decision-making model in its Code of Ethics.

Several models have been proposed to facilitate ethical decision making across psychological specialties, some of which built upon the five steps identified by Knapp and VandeCreek (2003) to provide a more comprehensive and detailed conceptual framework (e.g., Bush, 2007; Bush, Connell, & Denney, 2006; Hanson, Kerkhoff, & Bush, 2005; Knapp, Gottlieb, & Handelsman, 2015; Martin & Bush, 2008). Specific to geriatric mental health, Bush offered a 10-step model designed to promote ethical decision making for clinicians working with older adults. In contrast to the detailed model offered by Bush, Karel (2011) provided a more streamlined model that consists of five steps. We believe that integrating these two models covers the components of ethical decision making in a comprehensive manner without becoming overly detailed. Exhibit 3.2 describes this ethical decision-making process designed to aid geropsychologists in avoiding ethical misconduct and pursuing ethical ideals. A mnemonic for the process, CORE OPT, may facilitate its retention and recall. Practitioners might find that some steps in the model can be combined (e.g., by soliciting information on related areas as part of a single step).

Resources

Ethical decision making requires geropsychologists to ask and answer the question "What should I do?" To answer the question, geropsychologists must first decide, "What information do I need to make a good decision?"

EXHIBIT 3.2
CORE OPT: Model for Ethical Decision Making in Geropsychology

Clarify the ethical issue
Obligations owed to stakeholders
Resources (ethical and legal)
Examine personal beliefs and values

Options, solutions, and consequences
Put plan into practice
Take stock, evaluate outcome, and revise as needed

Psychological science, the evidence it generates, and the resources that compile and present the evidence underlie clinical decision making. As with clinical decision making, reviewing and considering relevant resources facilitates ethical decision making. The Ethics Code (APA, 2010) notes the value that can be obtained from considering multiple authoritative resources. In the Introduction and Applicability section, the Code states,

> In applying the Ethics Code to their professional work, psychologists may consider other materials and guidelines that have been adopted or endorsed by scientific and professional psychological organizations and the dictates of their own conscience, as well as consult with others within the field.

The following resource types promote ethical decision making:

- jurisdictional laws;
- professional ethics codes, particularly the APA Ethics Code (2010);
- *Code of Conduct* (Association of State and Provincial Psychology Boards, 2013);
- ethics committees, stated licensing boards, and liability insurance carriers;
- position papers of professional organizations;
- scholarly publications;
- institutional guidelines and resources; and
- informed and experienced colleagues.

Use of such resources reduces reliance on subjective impressions. Geropsychology endorses the scientist–practitioner, scholar–practitioner, and clinical science models of education, training, and practice, each differentially highlighting the relative value of available empirical evidence to inform clinical decisions. However, in the context of ethical decision making, there is a tendency to revert to "I think" solutions. For example, when colleagues are asked for advice about handling ethical challenges, it is not uncommon for the advice to begin with "I think you should . . ." A gold standard reply to a complex ethical question would begin with a statement such as "Based on ethical standard X, state law Y, position paper Z, my clinical experience, and my knowledge of how you feel about such issues, an appropriate course of action would be. . . ." Such an evidence-based approach to ethical decision making is more consistent with rational and systematic therapeutic decision making.

To further illustrate this point, consider the case of an older adult who is brought by her daughter for an evaluation of her financial decision-making capacity. The competent geropsychologist does not simply rely on the patient's daughter's account of the problems to make a diagnosis and determination about decision-making capacity. Instead, the geropsychologist conducts a thorough interview of the patient and her daughter, observes the patient, performs or refers for cognitive and psychological testing, integrates the information obtained from these various sources, considers all diagnostic possibilities, reviews relevant literature and consults with colleagues as needed, and then offers impressions.

Although many ethical and legal resources consist of principles and guidelines that are based on shared values of a society or profession, some resources have an empirical basis that further strengthens the guidelines. Studies of the effects of third-party presence during cognitive testing provide a good example of how empirical research informs ethical and professional decision making. (See the special issue of the *Journal of Forensic Neuropsychology*, edited by McCaffrey, Lynch, & Yantz, 2005.) Geropsychologists are best prepared to make sound ethical decisions when they maintain familiarity with core resources over the course of their career, rather than attempting to gather and understand the resources while in the middle of a crisis.

Application of General Bioethical Principles in Geropsychology

General bioethical principles are typically used by medical and mental health professions to guide the behavior of their members. Use of a common philosophical system allows for shared understanding that facilitates interdisciplinary communication regarding ethical matters. Beauchamp and Childress (2013) described four core biomedical ethical principles: respect for autonomy, nonmaleficence, beneficence, and justice.

Respect for autonomy refers to the right of competent, informed adults to make the decisions that govern their lives, as long as the decisions do not have negative effects on the rights of others. The principle underlies the right of patients to accept or decline examination or treatment and to be included in the medical decision-making process. This principle stands in contrast to the paternalistic approach traditionally applied in medicine whereby clinicians assume that they know which health care decisions and interventions are in the patient's best interests. Often, because of the nature of the setting and context in which services are provided or because of ageist assumptions, the rights of older adult patients to self-determination are overlooked or given secondary consideration. In the implied interest of expediency, decisions are often made for older adults with services administered to them, rather than inviting older adult patients to be partners in choosing and designing their assessment and treatment programs. Older adults, like younger patients, base health care decisions on their personal values, which may be shared with or different from the geropsychologist's values (Whitlatch, Feinberg, & Tucke, 2005). As detailed in Chapter 4, "mapping" and highlighting the divergent values of older patients and their loved ones and treating health care professionals may assist with reconciling differences in long-term care decision making (McCullough, Wilson, Teasdale, Kolpakchi, & Skelly, 1993). All parties benefit when geropsychologists strive to understand their patients' core personal values while maintaining an awareness of their own beliefs and values and the potential impact of their values on their clinical actions and decisions. This principle is reflected in the APA (2010) Ethics Code in Principle E (Respect for People's Rights and Dignity).

The principle of *nonmaleficence* reflects the classic mandate to do no harm. Despite seeming obvious on its surface, making decisions in individual cases about which action or inaction constitutes harm or to which patient, institution, or system the principle applies can prove quite challenging. The related principle of *beneficence* refers to a moral obligation to strive to promote patient welfare. Beneficence encompasses the advancement of the rights and health of others, defense of the rights of others, and prevention of harm. For example, a geropsychologist may encourage a patient who was recently admitted to a palliative care unit to perform a life review and record it for future generations, believing that such an activity would promote the psychological adjustment of the patient (beneficence); however, upon encountering emotional distress and resistance to the idea, the geropsychologist determines that the patient is not ready to accept his imminent death and that such a potentially therapeutic activity would be emotionally harmful to this patient at this time, so the activity is postponed (nonmaleficence). These two principles are captured in the Ethics Code in Principle A (Beneficence and Nonmaleficence).

The principle of *justice* reflects the availability and provision of fair, equitable, and appropriate treatment based on what patients are due or owed (Beauchamp & Childress, 2013). Distributive justice and formal justice are two distinct types. *Distributive justice* refers to the equitable distribution of health care or mental health resources. *Formal justice* refers to equal treatment for those who are equals and differential treatment for those who are not equals. Determining what is equitable and which individuals or groups are equals challenges clinicians in their application of this principle in the unique contexts in which ethical decision making is needed. The importance of both types of justice is reflected in the Veterans Affairs' (VA) home-based primary care (HBPC) program, which is essential for many older veterans because of their limitations with mobility and transportation. Through the HBPC program, the VA provides health care and mental health services for those veterans who are unable to travel to a VA facility, just as it does for those who can travel (distributive justice), while not using its resources for those who do not qualify for veterans benefits (formal justice). Outside of the VA system, distributive justice may be particularly problematic for geropsychologists practicing in rural or remote areas, frequently listed as mental health shortage areas (Institute of Medicine, 2012). This principle is captured in the Ethics Code in Principle D (Justice).

Two additional moral principles, fidelity and general beneficence, have been described as applicable to mental health professionals (Knapp & VandeCreek, 2006). *Fidelity* reflects the psychologist's obligation to be truthful and faithful, keep promises, and maintain loyalty. Although this principle may seem obvious, application in some contexts may not be easy or straightforward for geropsychologists. For example, an older adult patient in a subacute rehabilitation facility may request an urgent session with the geropsychologist. The geropsychologist is not able to see the patient at the time requested and, after assessing that there is no risk of danger, promises the patient that she will see the patient that afternoon. However, at the appointed time, the geropsychologist is handling an "administrative crisis," and by the time she is available, the patient has gone to physical therapy, which lasts until the time the geropsychologist leaves for the day. Thus, the geropsychologist did not keep the promise to see the patient that day, and her loyalty to the patient seems to have been sacrificed to her loyalty to the facility. Thus, geropsychologists must consider their ability to keep promises prior to making them and be clear and truthful about commitments when loyalties conflict. This principle is reflected in the APA Ethics Code in Principle B (Fidelity and Responsibility) and Principle C (Integrity).

General beneficence refers to the clinician's responsibility to the public at large (i.e., society). As an example, Knapp and VandeCreek (2006) described the responsibility of psychologists to protect future consumers of psychological evaluation services by safeguarding the integrity of psychological tests. Widespread availability of psychological test questions and responses threatens the validity of the measures for use with those who have been exposed to the measures, which could result in inaccurate diagnoses, unnecessary and potential harmful treatments, and misallocation of benefits (Bush & Martin, 2006). Despite the importance of this issue (i.e., test security), this example may be more reflective of avoidance of harm (nonmaleficence) than the promotion of benefit per se. Having a general obligation of beneficence to persons we do not know is a complex and controversial issue (Beauchamp & Childress, 2013), and its application should be carefully considered with individual cases and situations.

In the context of geriatric medicine and long-term care, and with the general biomedical ethical principles (Beauchamp & Childress, 2013) as the foundation, Feinsod and Wagner (2007) presented 10 ethical principles. Principles such as "futility of treatment" and "nonabandonment" further delineate the geropsychologist's ethical and professional responsibilities. *Futility of treatment* refers to the need for geropsychologists to modify or discontinue services when patients are not benefiting. With some older adult patients, psychotherapy sessions may seem more like "friendly visits" that the patients enjoy but that provide little, if any, benefit above what a visit from an untrained volunteer would provide. While patients may appreciate and value the visits, clinicians have a responsibility to consider whether such sessions reflect evidence-based care and advance patients toward attainment of therapeutic or functional goals; if not, changes or termination may be indicated. It is imperative that the geropsychologist carefully consider the equipoise of futility of treatment and nonabandonment within the context of the older person's economic circumstances in potentially ambiguous cases. It is also true, however, that even cognitively compromised patients who do not understand the geropsychologists may benefit from behavioral treatment plans, family interventions, or other services, and in such instances the interventions, by enhancing the patient's well-being, maintaining meaningful engagement, or improving the residential milieu, are far from futile. Geropsychologists who practice in interdisciplinary clinics, training clinics, or long-term care settings may provide such services at no or low cost, potentially changing the balance between futility of treatment and nonabandonment considerations.

The principle of *nonabandonment* reflects the importance of maintaining or otherwise facilitating appropriate care that benefits and is not harmful to patients. This principle helps guide clinicians through the often gray area between appropriate termination or transfer of treatment and the neglectful ending of psychological services. Geropsychologists may want to terminate treatment after becoming discouraged or frustrated with a patient or patient's family for a variety of reasons, including a lack of compliance with care or challenging, threatening, or intrusive personality traits. Geropsychologists may discontinue services in a reasonable time frame after resources have been provided to either the patient or a proxy to facilitate an appropriate transition of care. To address conflicts between clinicians and patients or their proxies, the guidance or assistance of an ombudsman, ethics committee, Department of Health official, or other appropriate resource can facilitate an acceptable resolution. General bioethical principles provide valuable direction for professional behavior. The principles are particularly valuable for establishing a good course of action when the Ethical Standards of the Ethics Code do not provide the needed direction or conflict with each other or with jurisdictional laws. However, the biomedical ethical principles can conflict with each other as well. When that occurs, the ethical decision-making model (Exhibit 3.2), becomes particularly helpful in answering the question "What should I do?"

Application of Psychological Ethics in Geropsychology

The Ethics Code's General Principles and Ethical Standards provide core information for the ethical practice of psychology. Although the standards are only enforceable for members of APA or in jurisdictions in which the governing body for psychologists has adopted them for their rules of conduct, the code is a valuable resource for all psychologists striving to engage in ethical practice. Depending on one's practice context and specific patient population, different components of the code take on greater or lesser importance. For example, a geropsychologist providing therapeutic services in a long-term care facility as part of a private practice and a university-based geropsychologist conducting research on the benefits of computerized mental exercises for healthy, high-functioning older adults will find different aspects of the code more relevant for their professional activities. Geropsychologists have a responsibility to understand those aspects of the code that are most relevant to their specific practice activities, aware that different standards may apply in individual cases. Additionally, because of the diverse practice opportunities available to geropsychologists and the increased risk of ethical misconduct when transitioning between practice settings or activities, there is a responsibility to become familiar with the most relevant ethical issues and legal requirements of the contexts in which geropsychologists anticipate working. Because the code is not intended to provide specific direction for psychological specialties such as geropsychology, supplemental resources are particularly valuable for specialists.

PROFESSIONAL GUIDELINES

A variety of documents published by professional organizations provide direction for geropsychologists. The following list includes some of the key guidelines for geropsychologists (see Bush, 2009, for a more comprehensive list of interdisciplinary guidelines that are relevant to geriatric mental health).

- *Assessment of Older Adults With Diminished Capacity: A Handbook for Lawyers* (American Bar Association Commission on Law and Aging & APA, 2005)
- *Assessment of Older Adults With Diminished Capacity: A Handbook for Psychologists* (American Bar Association/APA Assessment of Capacity in Older Adults Project Working Group, 2008)
- *Judicial Determination of Capacity of Older Adults in Guardianship Proceedings* (American Bar Association, APA, & National College of Probate Judges, 2006)

- *Making Treatment Decisions for Incapacitated Elderly Patients Without Advance Directives* (American Geriatric Society Ethics Committee, 2002)
- *Guidelines for the Evaluation of Dementia and Age-Related Cognitive Change* (APA, 2012a)
- *Guidelines for Psychological Practice With Older Adults* (APA, 2014c)
- *Pikes Peak Model for Training in Professional Geropsychology* (Knight et al., 2009)

Because position statements and other guidelines are drafted by professionals from different organizations or within the same organization at different points in time, there can be differences in perspectives or interests that result in conflicting recommendations. When they encounter such discrepancies, geropsychologists should investigate where and how opinions from multiple resources converge, with an appreciation that some resources carry more weight than others for given issues.

A seminal document for geropsychologists, the APA (2014c) *Guidelines for Psychological Practice With Older Adults*, provides 21 guidelines that span six broader categories: (a) competence in and attitudes toward working with older adults; (b) general knowledge about adult development, aging, and older adults; (c) clinical issues; (d) assessment; (e) intervention, consultation, and other service provision; and (f) professional issues and education. These guidelines "are intended to assist psychologists in evaluating their own readiness for working with older adults and in seeking and using appropriate education and training to increase their knowledge, skills, and experience relevant to this area of practice" (APA, 2014c, p. 34). The authors noted that the guidelines "should not be construed as definitive and are not intended to take precedence over the judgment of psychologists," relevant laws, or APA policy or ethics (p. 34).

Consideration of Jurisdictional Laws

Laws play an essential role in determining appropriate professional behavior of geropsychologists. Many issues that are first thought of as reflecting professional ethics (e.g., informed consent, privacy and confidentiality, record keeping) are also addressed by jurisdictional laws. Laws governing the practice of geropsychology come from multiple sources, including court decisions, federal and state statutes (including psychology licensing laws and regulations), and the enforceable standards of the Ethics Code or the Association of State and Provincial Psychology Boards (2013) Code of Conduct if adopted by the state psychology licensing board. Experience suggests that many geropsychologists are more familiar with ethical requirements than the laws that govern the practice of psychology in general and practice with older adults specifically. This greater awareness of ethics is fortuitous because the Ethics Code is in many ways more conservative than laws, providing greater protection for patients and the public. However, unless the Ethics Code has been adopted by the state licensing board as psychology's legally mandated rules of professional conduct in the state, violation of the code can result in censure by, or expulsion from, the APA, whereas violations of law can result in even greater penalties such as the loss of one's license to practice and criminal prosecution. Regardless of the potential consequences, all parties benefit when geropsychologists are familiar with both the ethics and laws that govern their practices.

Like state laws, a number of federal laws protect the rights of older adults who receive geropsychological services. While those laws that apply to the care of younger adults are also relevant for older adults, additional laws specifically address the care and well-being of older adults. The Older Americans Act, first passed in 1965 and most recently amended and reauthorized in 2006 (U.S. Department of Health and Human Services, Administration on Aging, 2006), reinforces the value of dignity as an inherent right of older adults, establishes entitlements to which older adults must have an equal opportunity for full and free enjoyment, and tasks the U.S. government with duties and responsibilities to promote the dignity of older Americans. The entitlements covered by the Older Americans Act include (a) access to the best possible physical and mental health services; (b) restorative care in institutions and maintenance services in the home, including family and caregiver support; (c) immediate benefits of proven research knowledge that can sustain and improve health and happiness; (d) autonomy in planning and managing their own lives; and (e) protection from abuse, neglect, and exploitation (§3001). The clinical and ethical decision making of geropsychologists should include consideration of these freedoms and securities to which their patients are entitled.

Because aging is associated with increased medical problems that adversely affect cognitive and emotional functioning, the Americans With Disabilities Act (1990) is relevant for geropsychologists in a variety of service delivery contexts. The act was created to provide legislative support for the prevention of discrimination against people with disabilities (Beneficence) and for the promotion of participation in society by individuals with disabilities (Justice). The Americans With Disabilities Act addresses five areas: employment, public services, public accommodations, transportation, and telecommunications. Geropsychologists who consider the application of the Americans With Disabilities Act with their patients help promote adaptive functioning.

Federal legislation for financial matters, such as the Omnibus Budget Reconciliation Acts (OBRAs) of 1987 and 1989 and the Balanced Budget Act of 1997, has affected geropsychological services through its impact on common reimbursement sources. OBRA improved reimbursement by Medicare by raising reimbursement and eliminating the cap on the number of outpatient mental health sessions allowed. OBRA further addressed the inappropriateness of nursing homes serving as an alternative to psychiatric hospitals for older adults with serious mental illness, a trend that began with the movement to deinstitutionalize psychiatric inpatients (OBRA-87; U.S. Department of Health and Human Services, Office of the Inspector General, 2001). In an effort to improve care for all nursing home residents, OBRA also directed reductions in physical restraint use and promoted nonpharmacological means to address behavioral issues among nursing home residents. Through the OBRA, concerted efforts have been made to allow older adults with serious mental illness to remain in the least restrictive living environment, such as their own homes or other community settings (Olmstead v. L. C., 1999; Williams, 2000).

The Patient Self-Determination Act (PSDA; OBRA, 1990) became effective on December 1, 1991, and required health care institutions such as hospitals, home health care agencies, nursing homes, and hospices that receive federal funds such as Medicare to "educate" potential patients about their rights to make decisions about their own health care. Although not specific to older adults, the PSDA is very relevant to geropsychologists involved in assisting older clients and their families with advance care planning or planning for future health care or housing needs. The specific requirements of the PSDA are that individuals (a) have the right to facilitate their own health care decisions, (b) have the right to accept or refuse medical treatments, and (c) have the right to execute an advance directive. The PSDA also requires that institutions must inquire whether the individual has an advance directive and make note of the existence of such a document in medical records as well as educate staff and affiliates.

The Balanced Budget Act of 1997 established Medicare Part C (Advantage Plans) as a managed care option for those eligible for Medicare, but the program was never widely accepted, and the number of enrollees has declined over the years. Although these acts addressed some concerns of older adults with mental health needs, problems, confusion, and disagreement regarding some aspects of the acts persisted (see Reichman, Streim, & Loebel, 2004, for a review).

The Centers for Medicare and Medicaid Services (previously the Health Care Financing Administration) manages funding for medical and mental health services for many older adults. In that role, this agency has considerable influence on the regulation of mental health services, including coverage, quality indicators, and documentation. For example, a clear federal mandate exists for the detection and treatment of mental illness among residents of nursing homes (Health Care Financing Administration, 1992; Reichman et al., 2004); however, the mandate does not mean that competent psychological services can be accessed and made available (Colenda et al., 1999; Reichman et al., 1998). Federal funding through the VA also supports psychological care for a large number of older adult veterans and their spouses. Geropsychologists who practice within such facilities or systems should be familiar with the regulations that govern their practices.

According to the U.S. Department of Health and Human Services, Administration for Community Living, Administration on Aging (2015), the Patient Protection and Affordable Care Act of 2010 (i.e., Affordable Care Act) provides new opportunities for older adults, their caregivers, and individuals with disabilities by (a) providing better care by aligning medical care with easily accessible, participant-centered home and community-based supports and services; (b) promoting improved health through education, assessment, disease prevention, and health promotion programs; and (c) lowering costs through efficient high-quality services, payment system reform, and fraud education and prevention. The law reportedly strengthens Medicare and provides new benefits and services to beneficiaries; increases incentives to enhance coordination between hospitals, physicians, and community service providers; creates the new Medicare-Medicaid Coordination Office to coordinate efforts between the programs and across federal agencies, states, and stakeholders; invests in innovation; supports community and clinical prevention services; and strengthens public health infrastructure.

The Health Insurance Portability and Accountability Act of 1996 (HIPAA) is a federal statute that regulates the manner in which patient information is maintained, used, and disclosed (U.S. Department of Health and Human Services, 2003). Among its features, the law promotes the privacy and security of patient information, and it affords patients the right to review and correct their health care information. Despite the importance of family involvement in the health care of many older adults and the benefits of openly sharing information, clinicians should not assume that all older adults, simply by virtue of their age, want their personal information shared with others. The desire for privacy is often maintained throughout one's life. Geropsychologists help maintain the privacy and integrity of patients by reminding themselves and other team members of the importance of determining with patients whether and with whom they want their medical information shared. It is not uncommon, however, for older adult patients in some medical settings to require care without being lucid enough to express their privacy wishes in advance. Staff members may need or want to communicate with family members; however, questions arise about whether they are permitted, because of HIPAA and other privacy laws, to do so under these circumstances. In such situations, health care professionals must balance the patient's health care needs with legal and ethical requirements, keeping in mind the best interests of the patient and consulting with institutional legal experts when appropriate.

Elder Abuse

Some older adults are abused, neglected, or exploited. The Older Americans Act of 1965 was designed, in part, to protect older adults from such mistreatment. The law has been amended every few years, most recently with the Older Americans Act Amendments of 2006 and the Older Americans Reauthorization Technical Corrections Act in 2007. State laws govern protection and reporting requirements, typically enforced through adult protective service agencies. However, the steps that psychologists should take when confronted with evidence of mistreatment or neglect of older adult patients vary by state.

In New York State, for example, psychologists are not legally mandated to report neglect or abuse of older adult patients simply because of their age. In the context of patient safety, health care providers are governed by the Family Protection and Domestic Violence Intervention Act of 1994. The Protective Services for Adults is the agency receiving and investigating reports of abuse of adults over the age of 18. Although it is not legally mandated to report maltreatment of older adults, there remains an ethical obligation to protect others. The first line of the first APA ethical principle (Principle A: Beneficence and Nonmaleficence) states, "Psychologists strive to benefit those with whom they work . . ." Although care must be taken to respect confidentiality rights, geropsychologists can often take a variety of steps to promote the welfare of abused, neglected, or exploited older adult patients that do not violate confidentiality, whether or not there is a legal mandate to report such maltreatment. Additionally, laws may exist to protect *vulnerable* patients of any age, and many older adults under the care of geropsychologists can be considered vulnerable persons. Geropsychologists need to be familiar with the laws governing reporting of maltreatment of older adult patients in their jurisdiction and decide on a course of action to take to protect vulnerable patients even in the absence of a mandate to report maltreatment.

Life-Sustaining Medical Care

Older adults confront declining health and serious medical procedures and are commonly asked for their preferences regarding life-sustaining care, such as artificial nutrition and hydration. Patients have a legal right to have such wishes respected (Cruzan v. Director, 1990; Patient Self-Determination Act, 1991; Washington v. Glucksberg, 1997). Health care facilities that receive Medicare and Medicaid funds must notify patients upon admission to the facility of their right to convey their preferences, including establishing advance directives. Courts have consistently placed a premium on patient self-determination and the importance of respecting autonomy in the context of terminal illness. For patients who have had artificial life-sustaining treatment initiated, they or their proxy have the legal right to discontinue the treatment, knowing that it will result in the patient's death. A distinction between withholding and withdrawing life-sustaining treatments has been rejected by courts (Barber v. Superior Court, 1983; Brophy v. New England Sinai Hospital Inc., 1986). Discontinuing feeding at the request of the patient or proxy is not considered suicide or active euthanasia but rather is viewed as allowing the underlying medical condition to follow its natural course (Reichman et al., 2004).

Conflicts Between Ethics and Legal Resources

Generally, professional ethics are consistent with legal requirements. However, there are situations in which conflicts are encountered between the laws under which geropsychologists practice, professional ethics, or beneficial clinical services. This situation is addressed in two places in the Ethics Code (APA, 2010). In the Introduction and Applicability section, the code states the following:

> In the process of making decisions regarding their professional behavior, psychologists must consider this Ethics Code in addition to applicable laws and psychology board regulations. . . . If this Ethics Code establishes a higher standard of conduct than is required by law, psychologists must meet the higher ethical standard. If psychologists' ethical responsibilities conflict with law, regulations, or other governing legal authority, psychologists make known their commitment to this Ethics Code and take steps to resolve the conflict in a responsible manner in keeping with basic principles of human rights.

Standard 1.02, Conflicts Between Ethics and Law, Regulations, or Other Governing Legal Authority, makes essentially the points.

In 1988, Pope and Bajt surveyed senior-level psychologists, including those knowledgeable about ethics, and found that 57% intentionally broke a law or a formal ethical standard at least once in consideration of client welfare or another deeper value. Knapp and colleagues (2007) stated, "These findings demonstrate that the guidance provided in Standard 1.02 is not sufficient in many cases and that ethical decision making is seldom as simple as we would like it to be" (p. 55). These authors provided a five-step question and answer process that helps clinicians clarify ethical and legal obligations and is likely to promote sound decision making when law, ethics, or values appear to conflict.

Perhaps the most important point is that anticipation of potential conflicts can help avoid problems from occurring.

In the context of HIPAA privacy requirements, Behnke, Perlin, and Bernstein (2003) stated, "At times HIPAA will preempt state law and at other times state law will preempt HIPAA" (p. 164). In such circumstances, geropsychologists must comply with the law that affords the patient greatest privacy.

Commitment to Positive Ethics and the Four A's of Ethical Practice

The term *positive ethics* may seem redundant if one considers that all professional ethics are designed to have a positive impact on professional behavior. Traditionally, however, ethics codes represent minimum professional standards and tend to be used primarily for remedial, disciplinary purposes. As reflected in the Ethics Code's General Principles, there is an ethical standard that is higher than the enforceable standards that is considered aspirational, thus optional. Rather than simply practicing in a manner that avoids ethical misconduct, *positive ethics* reflects a voluntary commitment to the pursuit of ethical ideals (Knapp & VandeCreek, 2012). A positive ethics approach requires a personal commitment to the highest standards of professional conduct.

Geropsychologists invested in such an approach to ethical practice make a conscious decision that a professional who strives for exemplary professional behavior represents the type of clinician that their patients, the public, and the profession deserve. Such an approach must be proactive, requiring geropsychologists to invest valuable time in considering ethical issues throughout their careers. The pursuit of ethical ideals is not without its challenges because it requires time and effort not expended by those more concerned with remedial ethics, but ethical conduct and patient welfare are maximized by the personal commitment to high standards of ethical practice and a proactive approach to ethical understanding and decision making. Appropriate standards of practice may be particularly vulnerable to compromise in forensic activities (e.g., decision-making capacity evaluations performed for attorneys) where there can be strong incentives or pressures to sacrifice objectivity or other standards of practice. A commitment to positive ethics can help geropsychologists avoid the moral disrepair that can result from sacrificing objectivity by essentially selling forensic opinions.

Positive ethics are facilitated by adherence to the four A's of ethical practice and decision making: anticipate, avoid, address, and aspire (Bush, 2009). Geropsychologists protect and promote patient welfare by (a) attempting to *anticipate* and prepare for ethical issues and challenges commonly encountered in their specific practice contexts, (b) striving to *avoid* ethical misconduct,

(c) taking steps to *address* ethical challenges when they are anticipated or encountered, and (d) maintaining a commitment to *aspire* to the highest standards of ethical practice. As Kerkhoff and Hanson (2015) reaffirmed, "ethical principles must be proactively, mindfully, and intentionally woven into daily practice in order for them to attain practical relevance" (p. 376).

CONCLUSION

The consistent ethical practice of geropsychology does not happen by accident; it takes work, and the work begins with a personal commitment to understand the relevant ethical issues and challenges, laws, and other guidelines that underlie appropriate professional behaviors. When anticipating or addressing ethical challenges, a systematic decision-making process that includes consideration of multiple resources is likely to facilitate the process. Pursuit of the highest standards of practice reflects a commitment to positive ethics, which promotes patient care. Being mindful of the four A's of ethical practice and decision-making positions geropsychologists to practice ethically and to model ethical behavior for students, trainees, other psychologists, and interdisciplinary colleagues.

II

FUNCTIONAL COMPETENCIES AND CASES

4

ASSESSMENT OF OLDER ADULTS

Don't become a mere recorder of facts, but try to penetrate the mystery of their origin.

—Ivan Pavlov

The quantitative and qualitative assessment of cognition, emotional state, behavior, and functional status in older adults is an essential task of geropsychologists, promoting appropriate decision making and clinical care. The assessment process is much broader than "testing" (Matarazzo, 1990), typically beginning with initial contact by the patient or a referral source and ending with a report that addresses (depending on the context) the referral question, other relevant findings, and recommendations. It is also common for treating clinicians to use standardized assessment measures to facilitate their treatment planning and monitor change over the course of treatment. Thus, some type of psychometric testing is commonly (but not always) a component of psychological assessment of older adults. Geropsychologists perform an assessment, not a testing. The primary goals of assessment are to facilitate understanding or well-being of the patient and to promote appropriate allocation of health care, support, and financial resources. These goals reflect the ethical principle of beneficence in clinical contexts and the principle of justice in both clinical

http://dx.doi.org/10.1037/0000010-005
Ethical Practice in Geropsychology, by S. S. Bush, R. S. Allen, and V. A. Molinari

and forensic contexts. Testing performed in isolation without a more comprehensive understanding of the older adult's background and current life context is at best very likely to be unhelpful; it is more likely to be misleading and harmful (Bush, 2014).

The assessment process consists of several components, which can be described broadly as (a) defining the referral question, (b) establishing and clarifying relationships, (c) obtaining informed consent or assent, (d) selecting and using procedures and measures, and (e) interpreting and documenting the findings. Additional steps are common, such as providing feedback to the patient, the patient's family or other representatives, and the referral source; presenting the findings to a court or other administrative or judicial decision maker; and monitoring the patient to ensure that treatment recommendations are implemented appropriately. Each step in this process brings unique ethical issues and potential challenges, as well as opportunities for clinicians who understand the ethical issues to provide beneficial services.

DEFINING THE REFERRAL QUESTION(S)

Overview

Geropsychologists evaluate older adults for many reasons, at the request of a variety of third parties; in addition, geropsychologists themselves may initiate the evaluation to better understand and monitor their own patients. Although the specific wording may vary widely, common referral questions typically seek to establish (a) psychiatric or neurocognitive diagnosis; (b) cause(s) of emotional, behavioral, or neurocognitive problems; (c) functional status and decision-making capacity; (d) prognosis; and (e) recommendations for treatment or care. Different practice settings and patient populations are likely to generate more of one type of referral question than another. Competent geropsychologists understand the types of referral questions that are most common in their practice settings but do not make unsubstantiated assumptions about referral questions for specific patients. Thus, an initial step in the assessment process is clarifying the goals and expected end product.

Vignette

A geropsychologist consulting in a skilled nursing facility receives a written referral to evaluate an 83-year-old man to "rule out pseudodementia." Having performed a number of evaluations with similar referral questions for the same referring physician and wanting to address the question quickly, the geropsychologist immediately performs the evaluation; finds that the patient is disoriented and has very poor attention but is not experiencing emotional distress; concludes that the patient does not have pseudodementia but does seem to be experiencing an acute delirium, likely resulting from an infection; documents the findings; and bills for his services. A week later the geropsychologist is confronted by the angry daughter of the patient, who complains that the evaluation was useless for her purposes, she will not pay the copay for the evaluation, and she may file complaints with the facility administration and Medicare because the evaluation, as performed, wasted valuable time and was unnecessary.

After asking for clarification, the geropsychologist learned that the patient's daughter, who is the patient's health care proxy, originally asked the consulting psychiatrist to assess whether the patient had financial decision-making capacity because she needed to take over her father's finances. The psychiatrist, seeking assistance, asked the attending physician to make a referral to the geropsychologist to help determine cognitive status and diagnosis. Unaware of the original reason for the evaluation, the attending physician submitted the referral for addressing such questions in the usual manner.

Ethical Decision-Making Process

As illustrated in Exhibits 3.1 and 3.2, a sequence of ethical decision-making questions and steps provides a structured approach to addressing ethical challenges. Asking oneself the questions and following the steps for each case is likely to help achieve good outcomes. When a working knowledge of the questions and steps has been achieved, they can often be addressed implicitly under conceptually integrated headings.

Ethical Issues, Tensions, and Resources

The geropsychologist has an ethical responsibility to provide services that benefit the patient, which include providing diagnostic clarification to the treatment team and facilitating other services or decisions that may be in the patient's interests. The ethical responsibility includes not performing services that are unnecessary or, through action or inaction, are harmful to the patient. To meet these responsibilities, the geropsychologist needs to clarify the reason for the evaluation and the uses to which the results will be put. Contacting the referral sources and engaging in an informed consent process with the patient's daughter would have provided the needed information.

The geropsychologist's attempt to be helpful by answering the referral question as quickly as possible (beneficence) conflicted with the need to avoid the potential harm (nonmaleficence) that could occur by acting too quickly and not being as thorough as needed to gather the requisite information about the reason for the referral.

Multiple sections of the *Ethical Principles of Psychologists and Code of Conduct* (APA, 2010; hereinafter, Ethics Code) are relevant. Principle A (Beneficence and Nonmaleficence) advises psychologists to "strive to benefit those with whom they work and take care to do no harm." Standard 3.04, Avoiding Harm, further establishes the need to take reasonable steps to avoid harming patients. Standard 3.07, Third-Party Requests for Services, requires psychologists to clarify with all involved parties at the outset of the service the probable uses of the services provided or information obtained. Standard 3.09, Cooperation with Other Professionals, requires psychologists, as needed, to cooperate with other professionals to serve their patients effectively and appropriately. Standard 3.10b, Informed Consent, states,

> For persons who are legally incapable of giving informed consent, psychologists nevertheless (1) provide an appropriate explanation, (2) seek the individual's assent, (3) consider such persons' preferences and best interests, and (4) obtain appropriate permission from a legally authorized person, if such substitute consent is permitted or required by law.

See also Standard 9.03, Informed Consent in Assessments.

The American Psychological Association (APA; 2012a) *Guidelines for the Evaluation of Dementia and Age-Related Cognitive Change* further describes the unique issues involved in the informed consent process with persons who are cognitively compromised (Guideline 3), with the psychologist striving to obtain all appropriate information for conducting the evaluation, including communicating with relevant health care providers (Guideline 6). The Standards for Educational and Psychological Testing (SEPT) stated, "These *Standards* presume that a legitimate . . . psychological . . . purpose justifies the time and expense of test administration. In most settings, the user communicates this purpose to those who have a legitimate interest in the measurement process . . ." (American Educational Research Association [AERA], APA, & National Council on Measurement in Education [NCME], 2014, p. 139).

Preferred Course of Action

The geropsychologist's evaluation would have been more useful and could have avoided angering the patient's daughter if the geropsychologist had contacted the referring physician upon receiving the referral, which would have led to clarification by the psychiatrist of the reason for the referral. Finding that the patient, in his delirium, lacked the cognitive capacity to provide informed consent for the assessment, the geropsychologist may have contacted the patient's health care proxy to get her consent, which would have provided further clarification of the reason for the assessment.

At this point, the geropsychologist could determine whether the actual reason for the referral could be answered by the information and data already obtained or whether additional assessment would be necessary, assure the patient's daughter that the matter would be addressed promptly, and consider performing the additional services at no additional charge.

ESTABLISHING AND CLARIFYING ROLES AND RELATIONSHIPS

Overview

It is often the case that multiple parties are involved in the psychological evaluation of older adults. Such parties include some combination of the following: the geropsychologist, other health care providers, the patient or examinee, the patient's family members or other caregivers, attorneys, administrative or legal decision makers, and facility administrators. Commonly, the various parties have different ideas about their roles and the roles of the others in the assessment process, and at times they may be unaware of the involvement of some of the other parties. For example, as illustrated in the first vignette of this book (see the Introduction), older adults are often brought for evaluations of cognitive and emotional functioning by their adult children, sometimes willingly and sometimes begrudgingly. In some instances, the person undergoing the evaluation and the person initiating the evaluation have different understandings of the purpose or nature of the evaluation or have competing goals for completing the evaluation. Establishing the relationships and ensuring that all known involved parties are clear about the relationships and everyone's role in the assessment process promotes a meaningful, rewarding, and beneficial assessment process for everyone involved.

Vignette

The adult son of a 65-year-old woman arranges an evaluation of cognitive and emotional functioning and personality changes for his mother. He reports that he has noticed significant changes in these areas, particularly with personality, over the past year or so. He states that he will be bringing his mother to the appointments, his sister will pay out of pocket for the evaluation, both of them want to be involved in providing background information, and he expects to be informed of the results. Upon initial interaction with the patient, there is no obvious indication that the patient has any cognitive deficits. During the informed consent process, when the limits of confidentiality are discussed, the patient refuses to have her children provide information about her or be informed of the results without her permission, which will depend on the findings.

Ethical Issues, Tensions, and Resources

The patient, a competent adult until evidence indicates otherwise, has the right to decide who will be involved in her evaluation and who will receive the results. However, the evaluation may be incomplete without the input of her close family members, potentially resulting in inaccurate and misleading results and inappropriate recommendations. The ability of the geropsychologist to conduct an assessment that is of value to the patient and her family (beneficence) requires access to all relevant information. The involvement of the patient's family is also required for logistical pur-poses as they are providing transportation and are funding the assessment. However, the patient's preference to not have family involved or informed of the results (respect for patient autonomy) conflicts with the requirements of an appropriate assessment.

Standard 3.07, Third-Party Requests for Services, states,

> When psychologists agree to provide services to a person or entity at the request of a third party, psychologists attempt to clarify at the outset of the service the nature of the relationship with all individuals or organizations involved. This clarification includes the role of the psychologist . . . an identification of who is the client, the probable uses of the services pro-vided or the information obtained, and the fact that there may be limits to confidentiality.

Geropsychologists clarify in advance who will receive the results and report (Standard 4.02, Discussing the Limits of Confidentiality). In the context of older adults specifically, because family members or others are often closely involved in the life, care, or decision making of the older adult patient, the geropsychologist should clarify with everyone involved (a) who the patient is; (b) the extent of involvement, if any, of the others; (c) the services that will be performed; (d) the extent and limits of privacy and confidentiality; and (e) the expected uses of information obtained and results generated.

Preferred Course of Action

The geropsychologist should call a family meeting or at least meet with the patient and her son to understand her children's interest in being involved and her reluctance to have them involved. The patient's children may be surprised to learn that the patient is concerned about them want-ing to have her "institutionalized," and she may be reassured to learn that her children are not interested in reducing her freedoms or taking over her finances but rather simply want her to get any care that might benefit her. The geropsychologist may assure the patient that the background information obtained from her children would be just one among many pieces of information that will be considered. If the patient remains reluctant to have the results shared with her children, she may accept a compromise of having the results conveyed to her primary medical doctor or sent to a neurologist as part of a more comprehensive work-up. Careful discussion and clarification with all involved parties at the outset of the services helps avoid uncertainty, inaccurate expectations, and conflict and can result in solutions that are satisfactory for everyone involved. When agreement cannot be reached and the geropsychologist believes that an assessment without such input would likely result in inaccurate findings, the assessment might be postponed, although a referral to another health care provider such as a neurologist or psychiatrist, which is commonly part of a thorough multidisciplinary assessment, can sometimes have a different result.

OBTAINING INFORMED CONSENT OR ASSENT

Overview

Competent adults have the right to make informed decisions about their health care, including whether to undergo recommended procedures or participate in recommended treatments. This right to be fully informed regarding health care services and to accept or decline participation based on that information is a legal right rooted in the Fourteenth Amendment Due Process provision of the U.S. Constitution, which states, "nor shall any state deprive any person of life, liberty, or property, without due process of law." Ethically, informed consent regarding proposed geropsychological services is reflected in the bioethical principle of Respect for Patient Autonomy and is described in multiple places in the APA Ethics Code.

In general, geropsychologists inform patients of the nature and purpose of the proposed services, fees, involvement of third parties, potential risks, and limits of confidentiality. Patients are also informed that there will be an opportunity for questions and discussion. The patient's involvement in all aspects of this process and decision should occur without excess influence by family members, health care professionals, or the geropsychologist.

> The first requirement for a valid legal consent is that the patient's participation in the decision-making process and the ultimate decision regarding care must be voluntary—without undue elements of force, fraud, deceit, overreaching, or other ulterior form of constraint or coercion. (Kapp, 2001, p. 24)

This informed consent process occurs as soon as possible in the clinical relationship and is carried out in formats (often oral and written) that are appropriate for the patient to ensure that the patient understands the information presented. Thus, "informed consent" is not simply a form to be completed, it is an interactive *process* between the geropsychologist and the patient that occurs as often as needed to ensure the patient's continued understanding of the issues covered.

Patients who clearly lack decision-making capacity, have questionable capacity to provide consent, or are mandated for services are nevertheless provided information about the nature and purpose of the proposed services, and it is generally respectful, clinically helpful, and ethically appropriate to seek the patient's assent (Standard 3.10b, Informed Consent; Standard 9.03b, Informed Consent in Assessments). In these situations the patient's willingness to participate in the assessment is still necessary for valid results to be obtained, and the patient, having been informed of the limits on confidentiality and the implications of failing to participate, may refuse. For individuals who have been deemed incompetent to make decisions regarding medical and mental health care and for whom a surrogate decision maker or guardian has been appointed, the surrogate's informed consent is needed for the proposed geropsychological services. In some settings, the surrogate consents to necessary testing and treatment when the patient is admitted to the facility. In all instances, the geropsychologist should be mindful of the rights and welfare of the patient when making decisions about possible services. Whether provided in a written or oral format, the consent process should be documented.

How Much Information to Disclose

Geropsychologists sometimes struggle with the question of how much information to disclose to patients during the informed consent process. Decisions about whether to provide detailed descriptions of the potential implications of undergoing a cognitive or psychological evaluation must be considered in the context of the patient's likelihood of refusing to undergo a potentially beneficial evaluation. Geropsychologists understand that some patients would refuse an evaluation if they fully understood that an abnormal result could jeopardize their normal freedoms. For example, when a cognitive assessment is recommended to determine a patient's capacity to manage medications, health care decisions, finances, or engage in daily activities such as cooking or driving, informing the patient that the results may be used as grounds for removal from the home or cessation of driving may result in a refusal to participate. However, the safety of the patient and others may depend on supervision or restriction of such activities, and the assessment results may be an essential component of the determination process.

Additionally, fully informed consent for an assessment may inter-fere with the ability of the geropsychologist to obtain valid test results, by discouraging patients from fully or accurately disclosing important background information and problems (J. M. Fisher, Johnson-Greene, & Barth, 2002). Similarly, understanding perceived negative ramifications of undergoing an assessment may heighten the patient's anxiety to a level that affects test performance. This situation involves a struggle between offering beneficial services and respecting the patient's right to decline the services; however, while the patient is granted the opportunity to accept or decline potentially beneficial services, the welfare of others in society may also hang in the balance. Providing general information about the purpose of the evaluation and immediate foreseeable risks, such as frustra-tion with difficult tasks, may satisfy informed consent requirements and maximize both the chances of the patient consenting to the assessment and the likelihood of valid results, but could be considered deceptive and a betrayal by some patients who subsequently lose freedoms, despite occur-ring in the interest of safety. From a practical perspective, it can be dif-ficult to determine in advance all the possible uses for assessment results, and attempting to do so would often lead to an unnecessarily detailed and lengthy informed consent process. Geropsychologists need to consider (in the context of a given assessment) the nature and extent of information, beyond the required minimum, conveyed to the patient to help with the decision-making process. The responsibility to err on the side of thorough-ness increases when the specific goal of the assessment is to assess abilities that affect safety.

Surrogate Decision Making

Situations arise in which patients are unable to make health care deci-sions for themselves or choose not to. In the context of geropsychological assessments, compromised decision-making capacity is the primary reason that a patient is unable to make such decisions. When patients are unable to make health care decisions, a surrogate, typically a family member, is selected or appointed to make the decisions, often based on advance directives such as living wills, powers of attorney, and health care proxies (Allen, Eichorst, & Oliver, 2013). It is the responsibility of the surrogate to be guided by the values and preferences of the patient when making decisions. There are two standards by which surrogate decisions are made: *substituted judgment* and *best interests*. Through substituted judgment, the surrogate strives to under-stand the patient's values and wishes to determine what decision the patient would make if it were possible for the patient to communicate effectively. This standard is favored by most courts and legislatures (Kapp, 2001). In the absence of an understanding or evidence about what the patient would decide, the surrogate bases decisions about services and care on what the surrogate believes would be in the patient's best interests. When the best interests standard is applied, there is a significant risk that surrogates will, intentionally or unintentionally, substitute their values and wishes for those of the patient. These issues, the types of decisions that can be made by surrogates, and the prioritizing of family members as surrogates are described in more detail in state statutes.

Usually, collaborative or shared decision making that involves the patient, surrogate, other family members, the geropsychologist, and other health care providers works well; however, contentious or anxious family members or surrogates who were not particularly close to the patient can make the process more challenging. Geropsychologists are well-suited to apply their knowledge and skills to educate and enable communication among all parties. Geropsychologists can sometimes facilitate the process by joining with the surrogate and other involved parties to create a values history for the patient. Similar to obtaining a medical and psychiatric history, obtaining a history of patients' values is often important for appropriate decision making. Unlike traditional advance directives, the values history provides an understanding of the patient as an individual rather than as a set of medical paradigms (Doukas & McCullough, 1991; Whitlatch, Feinberg, & Tucke, 2005). When taking a values history, the geropsychologist elicits information about the patient's lifestyle, life narrative, basic life values, and quality of life values, including attitudes and preferences regarding health, health care, and options for assessment, treatment, and comfort care.

Because of emotional involvement with the patient or other motivations, some surrogates may be tempted to make decisions that are inconsistent with the wishes previously conveyed by the patient. Examining their own values can help surrogates identify when their decisions represent their values rather than the patient's values and make decisions accordingly. Thus, obtaining values histories for patients *and* their surrogates can facilitate patients' wishes, except when surrogates intentionally act in their own interests. Some authors have provided forms to facilitate this process (Bush, 2009; Whitlatch et al., 2005). To further clarify and reconcile differences between the patient's and surrogate decision maker's values, geropsychologists may choose to obtain descriptions of the patient's values from at least two persons who knew the patient well prior to the cognitive decline. If discrepancies in their opinions exist, additional opinions should be sought from others.

From a cultural perspective, geropsychologists must be aware that in an increasingly diverse country and a world with rapidly expanding electronic communications, not all cultures share the Western commitment to autonomy. Working with patients' families and other health care providers to clarify patients' values and best interests is facilitated when geropsychologists are aware of, open to, and seek differences in understanding about what may be important to a given patient in the context of his or her ethnic group or dominant cultural identity.

Clinician Values

The ability of geropsychologists to identify their own values and separate them from the values of the patient promotes the patient's autonomy. Although one's personal values cannot, and perhaps should not, be removed entirely from ethically challenging situations, distinguishing between one's own values and those of the patient helps to clarify motives and results in a more reflective and potentially beneficial decision-making process. For example, with some patients, preserving independence may be worth accepting some level of substandard living or some risk of patient self-injury (Norris, Molinari, & Ogland-Hand, 2002). However, in other cases, such as when appointment of the surrogate decision maker or guardian is unresolved or the surrogate appears to be pursuing an agenda that is inconsistent with the best interests of the patient, it may be necessary for the geropsychologist to adopt a more traditional, paternalistic stance on the patient's behalf. Paternalism represents a protective, beneficent position that overrides the preferences of another (Beauchamp & Childress, 2013), which presents a conflict between beneficence and respect for patient autonomy. Considerable caution is indicated whenever geropsychologists, on the basis of their personal values or beliefs, consider interfering with a patient's right to make choices about important life issues. Any constraints on autonomy in the interest of beneficence must be supported by strong clinical evidence rather than conjecture (Macciocchi & Stringer, 2001). Because of the need to consider and prioritize state and federal laws, ethics codes, and other resources, clinicians may be well served by consulting legal counsel when adopting procedures and forms for informed consent and other practice-related issues.

Vignette

A 76-year-old man is brought to a geropsychologist's private practice office by his adult daughter who arranged the evaluation. The patient was informed by his daughter that the purpose of the evaluation was "just to make sure everything's all right with your memory," whereas the patient's daughter wants the geropsychologist to "do some tests and tell my father he can't drive anymore; he won't listen to me." She then informed the geropsychologist that her father would not undergo the evaluation if he knew that his ability to continue driving was on the line.

Ethical Issues, Tensions, and Resources

The patient may lack the ability to drive safely, placing him and others at risk of considerable harm. An evaluation of cognitive, sensorimotor, and psychological functioning could be an important part of a more comprehensive process of determining whether the patient should stop driving. Consistent with respect for patient autonomy and the informed consent process, the patient has a right to know the real purpose of the evaluation, including foreseeable risks and benefits, and to elect to participate or not. However, the patient's refusal to undergo the evaluation could put people's lives in danger. Alternatively, recommending that the patient be deprived of his freedom to drive could have a serious adverse effect on his quality of life and emotional state. The geropsychologist could promote the well-being of the patient (beneficence) and the society at large (general beneficence) by deceiving the patient regarding the purpose of the evaluation in order to potentially save lives, including the patient's. However, such deception could ruin any trust that the patient has in health care professionals and is typically inconsistent with ethical clinical services.

The desire to protect the patient and society (beneficence) conflicts with respect for the patient's right to make informed decisions about whether to undergo an evaluation by the geropsychologist (respect for patient autonomy). The Ethics Code (APA, 2010) states, "Psychologists establish relationships of trust with those with whom they work" (Principle B: Fidelity and Responsibility) and "seek to promote accuracy, honesty and truthfulness in the science, teaching and practice of psychology. In these activities psychologists do not steal, cheat or engage in fraud, subterfuge or intentional misrepresentation of fact" (Principle C: Integrity). However, Principle B also states that psychologists "are aware of their professional and scientific responsibilities to society and to the specific communities in which they work." Helping remove an unsafe driver from the road would be consistent with this principle and with the principle of general beneficence. Principle C addresses the issue of deception:

> In situations in which deception may be ethically justifiable to maximize benefits and minimize harm, psychologists have a serious obligation to consider the need for, the possible consequences of, and their responsibility to correct any resulting mistrust or other harmful effects that arise from the use of such techniques.

The Ethical Standards address deception in the context of research (Standard 8.07, Deception in Research) but not for clinical services.

In some assessment contexts, examiner deception is acceptable and in fact necessary. The assessment of symptom and performance validity involves use of measures that appear to be measuring one construct (e.g., memory) when they are actually measuring another construct (e.g., engagement in the testing process, effort). Some of the tests have names that indicate they measure cognitive ability rather than test engagement, and some involve instructing the examinee that the test is particularly challenging when it is really extremely easy. In this context, psychologists use deception to detect possible deception, in the pursuit of an accurate understanding of the examinee's presenting problems. In the example of the older adult who perhaps should not be driving, deception would be used to possibly protect the patient and others. The standard of practice is to inform examinees that measures of effort and honesty (or some similar terms) will be used during the evaluation, but the specific validity assessment measures are not identified or described (Bush, Connell, & Denney, 2006).

Standard 3.10 (Informed Consent) states,

> (a) When psychologists . . . provide assessment . . . they obtain the informed consent of the individual or individuals using language that is reasonably understandable to that person or persons except when conducting such activities without consent is mandated by law or governmental regulation or as otherwise provided in this Ethics Code.

Standard 9.03, Informed Consent in Assessments, states more specifically,

> (a) Psychologists obtain informed consent for assessments, evaluations or diagnostic services, as described in Standard 3.10, Informed Consent, except when (1) testing is mandated by law or governmental regulations; (2) informed consent is implied because testing is conducted as a routine educational, institutional or organizational activity (e.g., when participants voluntarily agree to assessment when applying for a job); or (3) one purpose of the testing is to evaluate decisional capacity. Informed consent includes an explanation of the nature and purpose of the assessment, fees, involvement of third parties and limits of confidentiality and sufficient opportunity for the client/patient to ask questions and receive answers.

For the geropsychologist, the purpose of the assessment becomes the center of the ethical dilemma, as it can be defined in various ways. The purpose of the assessment could be conceptualized and described along the following lines: (a) to determine cognitive strengths and weaknesses; (b) to determine the presence and nature of a neurocognitive disorder, if any; (c) to determine whether safety is affected by cognitive deficits; (d) to make a recommendation regarding ability to drive; or (e) to address some combination of these or other purposes. Although all of the purposes would be accurate, the choice of which purpose is presented to the patient would likely determine whether he would participate. Only one purpose would be likely to trigger a refusal to participate.

"Informed consent is decidedly the starting point for the patient–provider relationship" (Johnson-Greene & the NAN Policy & Planning

Committee, 2005). When most successful, informed consent is a collaborative process of shared decision making in which mutually agreed-upon goals are identified and the manner in which the goals will be pursued is specified (Knapp & VandeCreek, 2006). Standard 8.2 of the *Standards for Educational and Psychological Testing* states the following:

> Test takers should be provided in advance with as much information about the test, the testing process, the intended test use, test scoring criteria, testing policy, availability of accommodations, and confidentiality as is consistent with obtaining valid responses and making appropriate interpretations of test scores. (AERA, APA, & NCME, 2014, p. 134)

Standard 8.4 states,

> Informed consent implies that the test takers or their representatives are made aware, in language that they can understand, of the reasons for testing, the types of tests to be used, the intended uses of test takers' test results or other information, and the range of material consequences of the intended use. (p. 134)

Given the very narrow scope and questionable appropriateness of the presenting referral question, working with the patient's daughter at the outset to more appropriately conceptualize and broaden the purpose of the evaluation may better serve the patient and his daughter.

In its publication *A Physician's Guide to Assessing and Counseling Older Drivers*, the American Medical Association (2009) described ethical and legal considerations, with a focus on reporting requirements and their effect on patient confidentiality.

> The need for patient confidentiality cannot be considered absolute; a patient is entitled to freely disclose his or her symptoms and condition to his or her physician in confidence except where the public interest or the private interest of the patient so demands, and thus a patient possesses a limited right to patient confidentiality in extra-judicial disclosures subject to exceptions prompted by the supervening interest of society. (p. 60)

It is concluded that patient confidentiality does not necessarily protect doctors from their nondisclosure in cases of driving-impaired patients. Clinicians should recommend that unsafe drivers cease driving if their driving cannot be made safe by medical treatment, adaptive devices, or adaptive techniques. Such recommendations should be based on the patient's driving abilities rather than the patient's age, should include a system for checking on future compliance, and should be documented in the patient's chart.

In balancing the principles of beneficence and respect for patient autonomy, Beauchamp and Childress (2013) described situations in which a paternalistic stance that decreases patient autonomy is justified and even necessary. They distinguished between *soft* and *hard* paternalism. In their discussion of soft paternalism, the authors stated, "Preventing minor harms or providing minor benefits while deeply disrespecting autonomy lacks plausible justification, but actions that present major harms or provide major benefits while only trivially disrespecting autonomy have a plausible paternalistic rationale" (p. 221). In contrast, even hard paternalism, which infringes more significantly on patient autonomy, is justified in the following situations: (a) a patient is at risk of a significant, preventable harm; (b) the paternalistic action will probably prevent the harm; (c) the prevention of harm to the patient outweighs risks to the patient of the action taken; (d) there is no morally better alternative to the limitation of autonomy that occurs; (e) the least autonomy-restrictive alternative that will secure the benefit is adopted; and (f) the paternalistic stance should not damage substantial autonomy interests (e.g., religious or cultural practices that do not harm others). In the specific context of "older adults who are, or are at risk of becoming, impaired drivers," Knapp and VandeCreek (2005) argued that "concern for patient and public welfare caused by driving impairments may sometimes override respect for patient autonomy" (p. 197).

Some states have addressed, either by statute or common law, the obligations of doctors to report to drivers' licensing authorities when a patient's driving abilities have become impaired by age-related neurodegenerative illness or sensory deficits (Kapp, 2001). In some of these states, the clinician is mandated to report patients who have a medical condition that might be hazardous to driving even when determining driving ability was not a goal of the assessment. California specifically requires physicians to report all cases of diagnosed Alzheimer's disease and related disorders (California Health & Safety Code §1039009; see also Family Caregiver Alliance, 2001). In states with mandating reporting laws, failure to comply could result in professional discipline, and civil damages may be pursued even in the absence of such laws (Kapp, 2001). Even in states without mandatory reporting laws, clinicians may not face penalties for breaking confidentiality to report unsafe drivers when acting in good faith and instead may be held liable for failing to report unsafe drivers (American Medical Association, 2009). Knowledge of current laws in the jurisdiction in which the clinician practices is essential.

> Laws, regulations and policies vary not only by State but also by local jurisdiction, and are subject to change. Therefore, it is important for physicians to seek out legal advice from a licensed attorney in their States on specific issues or questions that may arise with an individual patient. (American Medical Association, 2009, p. 59)

Preferred Course of Action

Initial interaction with a patient or the person contacting the geropsychologist on behalf of the patient provides an opportunity for the geropsychologist to gather preliminary information about the reason for the contact so that a decision can be made about whether or which services are needed. When the geropsychologist was contacted by this patient's daughter and the reason for the requested evaluation was explained, the geropsychologist had the opportunity to ask about any collisions, "close calls," or problems that the patient has had while driving or in other aspects of his life (e.g., frequent falls, forgets to turn off the stove) that may provide initial insight into current functioning ability. Such information can help the geropsychologist anticipate the deficits that may be encountered and prepare a good approach to the informed consent process; care should be taken to avoid the anticipatory bias that can result in inaccurate diagnoses and inappropriate recommendations.

During the informed consent process, the geropsychologist can inform the patient that the cognitive testing is indeed intended to determine how well he is doing with memory, attention, spatial abilities, sensory and motor functions, and other abilities that will be assessed, and that such testing is done to help promote safety. The results of the evaluation might cause the geropsychologist to determine that the patient has extremely slow speed of processing and reaction time and poor spatial skills and should not be driving or should undergo a more formal driving evaluation before continuing to drive; in that case, she should explain that to the patient in a feedback session, and she should be prepared to address any "mistrust or other harmful effects that arise" from the recommendations (see APA [2010] Ethics Code, Principle C: Integrity). In some states, the geropsychologist may have a legal obligation to make a report to the department of motor vehicles, which could result in the patient's feeling a strong sense of betrayal. In such instances, addressing a patient's adverse emotional reaction to such information includes use of basic humanistic therapy techniques (i.e., empathy, genuineness, unconditional positive regard) combined with education about why such recommendations were made or actions taken (Cain, Keenan, & Rubin, 2015). Sometimes, use of a concrete example can drive home the point. An example might be along the lines of the following exchange:

Geropsychologist: You have grandchildren, right?

Patient: Yes, three granddaughters and a grandson.

Geropsychologist: How would you feel if you were driving home from the store one day, didn't react quickly enough to a changing stoplight, and hit a school bus full of children?

Patient:	That would be awful.
Geropsychologist:	Do you think it's worth the risk?
Patient:	I can't imagine not driving. But, no, it's not worth the risk.

SELECTING AND USING PROCEDURES AND MEASURES

Overview

Geropsychologists have at their disposal a variety of procedures and standardized assessment measures to facilitate an understanding of older adults. Use of such psychological measures is an essential part of the services provided to older adults. The results help clinicians establish treatment plans and monitor their effectiveness, and they provide others, including treatment team members, family members, and legal decision makers, objective evidence of cognitive, emotional, and behavioral functioning. The term *procedures* encompasses a broad range of activities, such as interviews, observations, record reviews, and testing. Clinical interviews typically precede testing because the information gained from the interaction assists the geropsychologist with selecting appropriate measures to meet the unique needs of a given patient. Interviews of the patient and collateral sources of information also provide essential information on the older adult's functional capacity in his or her social and physical environment (APA, 2014c).

The term *measures* refers to tests, most of which are standardized and objective. Geropsychologists' use of objective, standardized measures with appropriate normative bases provides a particularly unique and valuable contribution to the understanding and care of older adults. In some contexts, such as rural and low resource areas where educational and health disparities exist, the establishment of local norms may further help geropsychologists to obtain an accurate understanding of patients' strengths and weaknesses. Because of regional variability in responses to some questions or performance on certain tasks, developing normative data that reflect the characteristics of the local population can allow for comparisons that are more representative of the person being assessed regarding the constructs of interest. Using local norms can help avoid the overpathologizing of patients that can occur when comparing them with national norms that may be more stringent. (The use of national norms may be preferred depending on the purpose and nature of the assessment; geropsychologists use their understanding of the relevant issues when selecting norms for a given patient.)

Whether to use psychometric instruments and, if so, which tests to use are critically important decisions in the assessment of older adults. Many tests that were developed and standardized with younger populations lack or have insufficient normative data for older age ranges, particularly with diverse populations. When such measures are used with older adults, their validity is compromised. Additionally, some measures or batteries that are lengthy may be too taxing for some older adults so that fatigue, rather than deficits with the construct of interest, negatively affects performance. However, brief screening measures often lack sensitivity to relatively subtle cognitive deficits. Although computerized and online testing are being used with increased frequency, geropsychologists should be mindful that older adults, as a group, tend to be less familiar with computers, and the prospect of being judged on the basis of performance on such an unfamiliar device can trigger considerable anxiety in some older adult patients. Prior to administering computer-based tests, geropsychologists should determine the patient's comfort level with such technologies; be prepared to offer alternate, traditional test administration options; and describe any impact that computerized administration may have had on the test results (Browndyke, 2004; Schatz, 2004).

With measures of emotional state, the nonspecific nature of some of the items can result in their endorsement because of physical rather than affective problems, raising unwarranted concerns about the patient's emotional state. Because some older adults have sensory or motor deficits that interfere with standardized test administration, usual administration procedures may need to be modified to allow an adequate sample of behavior, ability, or emotional state to be obtained. For these reasons, careful selection and use of assessment measures are needed and should be tailored to the needs of the individual patient, based on the purpose of the assessment and with consideration of the assessment context.

Thorough assessments of older adults often involve a multimethod, preferably interdisciplinary approach. As stated in *Guidelines for Psychological Practice With Older Adults* (APA, 2014c), "A thorough geriatric assessment is preferably an interdisciplinary one" (p. 46). Edelstein and Koven (2011) noted, "It is the rare clinician who has the skills and knowledge to formally assess every facet of an older adult's functioning" (p. 56). Integrating information obtained from multiple measures and sources, including laboratory tests and neuroimaging, can maximize an understanding of the older adult's strengths and weaknesses and facilitate accurate diagnosis and appropriate care.

Because many older adults are accompanied to assessment appointments by family members or other caregivers, or the assessment is performed in an inpatient setting where others are commonly present, geropsychologists need to carefully consider whether a third party should or must be present during the assessment. A growing body of research has shown that the presence of third parties, including recording devices, affects examinee performance on cognitive and motor tests (see McCaffrey, 2005, for a review). As a result, professional organizations have advised against having third parties present during cognitive testing (American Academy of Clinical Neuropsychology, 2001; National Academy of Neuropsychology, 2000). In settings in which the presence of roommates or others during testing cannot be avoided, geropsychologists should strive to reduce the effects of their presence on the assessment process and consider, to the extent possible, the impact of their presence on the test results.

Vignette

A 92-year-old, African American woman who completed 7 years of education in a geographic area with known disparities in the quality of K–12 education is referred by her geriatrician for a psychological evaluation because her family reported that she has problems with memory. The patient lives with her daughter and is independent with daily activities. The psychologist interviews the patient and her daughter and then, because the patient is relatively high functioning and is evaluated on an outpatient basis, administers the Wechsler Adult Intelligence Scale—4th Edition (WAIS–IV; Wechsler, 2008), the Wechsler Memory Scale—4th Edition (WMS–IV; Wechsler, 2009), the Trail Making Test (Reitan & Wolfson, 1985), and Wisconsin Card Sorting Test (computer version; Heaton, Chelune, Talley, Kay, & Curtiss, 1993). The patient is compliant with the test but about halfway through begins to need prompting to keep trying her best because she seems to lose focus. Also, the psychologist must repeat questions and instructions multiple times to make sure the patient understands the material. Toward the end of the WMS–IV, the psychologist decides to modify test administration to accommodate the patient's apparent hearing problems by writing down the verbal response options and letting her select her choice by pointing. After test administration has been completed and the patient and her daughter leave, the psychologist realizes that he does not have demographically corrected norms for these tests for a 92-year-old, African American woman with 7 years of education. He decides to "extrapolate norms" from the next closest demographically correct norms and interpret the results "with caution."

Ethical Issues, Tensions, and Resources

The psychologist did not plan the assessment process, including test selection and administration, with the unique needs of this individual in mind. Because the psychologist wanted to conduct a comprehensive cognitive assessment that would be helpful to the patient (beneficence), his choice of tests was probably much more comprehensive than was necessary, which overly taxed the patient (nonmaleficence) and wasted time and resources (justice). Additionally, use of computerized tests with this patient may have induced anxiety or otherwise led to an invalid sample of her capabilities on some of the constructs of interest. There is also no indication in the vignette that the psychologist discussed the patient with her geriatrician or reviewed any medical records before administering the tests. What the psychologist believes to be poor comprehension may actually be hearing loss. Failure to attempt to learn more about the patient prior to meeting with her may have adversely affected the patient's test performance and biased the psychologist's conclusions and recommendations (nonmaleficence).

The primary ethical tension is between the principles of beneficence and nonmaleficence—that is, determining whether the benefits of the assessment for the patient outweigh the possible harm that could result from the strenuous process and potentially inaccurate conclusions. A process of moral deliberation and justification, informed by relevant resources, is needed to establish the preferred choice when such principles conflict (Beauchamp & Childress, 2013).

The process of choosing assessment measures begins by clarifying the purpose of the assessment and determining any unique characteristics of the patient that would influence choice of measures to be used to address the questions of interest (AERA, APA, & NCME, 2014; APA, 2014b). Standard 9.02, Use of Assessments, states,

> (a) Psychologists administer, adapt, score, interpret or use assessment techniques, interviews, tests or instruments in a manner and for purposes that are appropriate in light of the research on or evidence of the usefulness and proper application of the techniques. (b) Psychologists use assessment instruments whose validity and reliability have been established for use with members of the population tested. When such validity or reliability has not been established, psychologists describe the strengths and limitations of test results and interpretation. (APA, 2010)

Caplan and Shechter (2012) further clarified the relationship between the purpose of the evaluation and the selection and modification of tests:

> If the aim is to detect brain damage or dysfunction, there may be little need for other than pure, standardized administration of a test battery. If, however, what is sought is information about specific types of competence (e.g., cognitive "power" divorced from the need for speeded performance), performance-limiting and performance-enhancing factors and their implications for management, capacity to function safety, or a host of other possible referral questions, then what we have termed an "elastic" approach to the use of tests is often more fruitful. (pp. 109–110)

When considering whether to modify standardized testing procedures, geropsychologists strive to avoid unfair treatment of, and discrimination against, the patient (AERA, APA, & NCME, 2014).

Although standardized test administration is important for the accuracy and comparability of test score interpretations, there are situations in which departure from standardized procedures is necessary to gain some understanding of the construct of interest, although comparability may be sacrificed and the construct actually being assessed may depart to some degree from the construct that is assessed under standardized administration procedures (AERA, APA, & NCME, 2014). Caplan and Shechter (2012) identified six primary factors that warrant nonstandard modifications in the assessment of older adults: (a) patient unfamiliarity with the testing process; (b) diminished sensation; (c) fatigability; (d) behavioral slowing; (e) comorbid conditions, some of which affect motor functioning; and (f) medication effects, both positive and negative. Some empirical research exists to support specific modifications. For example, because some older adults sustain strokes that result in hemiparesis of their dominant side, they are unable to use their dominant hand to complete motor tasks and must instead use their nondominant hand. However, without empirical evidence to support use of the nondominant hand for such purposes, the appropriateness of comparing nondominant hand performance to normative data obtained with the dominant hand is questionable (Bush & Martin, 2004). Caplan and Shechter reviewed the literature on specific modifications, where they exist, across cognitive domains. They concluded that "assessment of the geriatric patient demands a high level of scientist–practitioner skill . . . the clinician benefits by being something of an artist–innovator" (p. 108).

The psychologist in this case also needed to consider cultural issues when reflecting on the nature of the assessment process and the measures to be used. The APA (2012a) *Guidelines for the Evaluation of Dementia and Age-Related Cognitive Change* state that psychologists take into account cultural issues and avoid engaging in discriminatory practice (Guideline 5). The guidelines further state: "Psychologists assessing older adults from racial and ethnic minorities strive to seek and use the best available tests for each individual's background and consult with expert colleagues as needed regarding interpretation" (Guideline 8, p. 5). As Byrd and Manly (2012) summarized,

> One consistent finding across cross-cultural studies of cognition in American ethnic groups is the existence of significant performance differences between neurologically healthy minority and Caucasian elders that persist after statistical corrections and matching for age, years of education and gender. (pp. 115–116)

These authors further noted that the performance differences, which result from multiple factors, result in a disproportionate number of misdiagnoses of neurocognitive disorders among minority elders. They described four sources of cultural effects on the neuropsychological test performance of older adults: (a) cultural experience; (b) quality of education, literacy, and years of education; (c) stereotype threat; and (d) unknowns, including the inadequacy of common tests to tap the complete range and potential of cognitive abilities in minority elders. In the specific context of test selection, Byrd and Manly stated,

> The clinician's choice of assessment measures is especially pertinent when evaluating culturally diverse elders . . . if the selected battery does not include measures that have been validated in the ethnic minority populations or that contain appropriate normative data, the clinician risks an invalid assessment. Evaluations with ethnic minority elders may require the clinician to alter their standard battery, especially if the client has limited education and/or minimal English language proficiency. (p. 118)

However, a primary challenge lies in the relatively limited, although increasing, availability of tests that have been developed and standardized with culturally diverse samples (Rivera Mindt, Arentoft, Coulehan, & Byrd, 2013).

The likelihood of patient fatigue during hours of cognitive testing and the effect on the patient's performance should also have been considered. As Woodard and Axelrod (2012) stated,

> The presence of fatigue that may develop during the assessment is also a major consideration in obtaining accurate assessment data . . . newer generation cognitive measures have focused on development of screening measures or brief administration times in order to mitigate this potential difficulty. (p. 73)

These authors specifically noted the potential dangers of fatigue affecting performance when the full version of the WAIS–IV is used. The impact of the time of day of the evaluation on a patient's level of arousal should also be taken into account because many older adults perform better on cognitive tasks earlier compared with later in the day.

Preferred Course of Action

Taking time in advance to learn more about the patient would have better positioned the psychologist to select more appropriate tests or design better modifications, thus allowing for the most accurate understanding of the constructs of interest and the patient overall. The psychologist also would have been well-served by consulting with a colleague who has more experience assessing African American older adults with a seventh-grade education from a geographic area with known educational disparities. The information provided by the colleague would likely have helped avoid pitfalls in the selection and use of assessment measures. Had the psychologist taken these steps, the potential for providing a beneficial assessment (beneficence) would probably have outweighed the likelihood that the assessment would be harmful to the patient (nonmaleficence).

INTERPRETING AND DOCUMENTING

Overview

The contribution of assessment to the understanding and care of the older adult is generated from the multistep, multimethod assessment process and is provided in the interpretation and reporting of the findings. An accurate, informative, and useful interpretation is based on competent performance of the preceding assessment steps; however, competence in the preceding steps does not ensure accuracy in the interpretation. Geropsychologists must integrate the various sources of information and data with their understanding of brain–behavior relationships, psychological functioning, medical disorders, effects of medications, measurement statistics, sources of measurement error, symptom and performance validity, cultural and social influences, and other factors that could have affected the information and data obtained. Having done that, the information must be applied to the specific purpose of the assessment in the specific context in which the assessment was performed. Finally, the manner in which the information is conveyed can affect its utility for the patient, referral source, and others. For example, brief concise verbal and written reports to a referring physician provided in everyday language may be more helpful than a lengthy, detailed, jargon-filled written report that is left in a patient's medical chart. Both the reporting process and the report content can make the assessment process useful or nearly useless, depending on how they are managed.

The evaluation of response, symptom, and performance validity is an integral part of the assessment process, and much has been written about it in recent years. Determining whether the patient responded honestly to interview and test questions and exerted an effort on ability tests is often the first step in the interpretation process. The evaluation of validity is often a multimethod process that includes both observational and psychometric components. Psychological tests, such as the Minnesota Multiphasic Personality Inventory (Hathaway & McKinley, 1943) and its revisions, have long included validity indices, and the numbers and types of validity scales continue to increase. Cognitive ability tests such as the Wechsler intelligence and memory scales now have empirically based indicators embedded within them to help evaluate performance validity. The same is true for some screening measures such as the Repeatable Battery for the Assessment of Neuropsychological Status (Randolph, 1998). Additionally, free-standing validity measures are available and commonly used.

Some psychologists who assess older adults have stated that empirical assessment of performance validity is unnecessary with older adults; others have claimed that they can tell when a patient is not trying. Unfortunately, research has shown that clinicians are not particularly good at determining, based solely on clinical judgment, when a patient's presentation is misleading or effort is suboptimal (see Guilmette, 2013). Additionally, failure to systematically consider validity issues simply because of the age of the patient is a form of ageism. Using empirically based measures to help determine the validity of test results is no less important for older adult patients than it is for younger patients. Professional organizations have taken the position that, except for very low-functioning patients, such as those requiring 24-hour care, psychometric assessment of performance validity is necessary in any medically necessary cognitive assessment (Bush et al., 2005; Heilbronner et al., 2009). Many reasons, other than malingering, might explain why older adults would not put forth good effort on cognitive tests; for example, they might be "forced" by their adult children, attorney, or primary medical doctor to undergo the assessment. Determining whether the test data are valid for interpretation is essential for avoiding diagnostic errors with older adults. Psychometrically based symptom validity tests (SVTs) and performance validity tests (PVTs) are commonly used to help determine whether the results of cognitive ability measures or psychological measures are valid for interpretation.

> It cannot be just assumed that anybody with a diagnosed serious neurological condition, including MCI or dementia, will put forth good effort during neuropsychological evaluations, so accurate assessment of symptom validity remains important. . . . At present, the consensus in the literature appears to be that the originally published cut-offs for many SVTs may not be applicable in cases of MCI or dementia, but with either adjusted cutoffs or actuarial profile analysis, specificity can be likely improved to acceptable ($\geq 90\%$) levels. (Donders & Kirkwood, 2013, pp. 402–403)

The maintenance and disclosure of records are based on jurisdictional laws (including protections in the Health Insurance Portability and Accountability Act, 1996), professional guidelines (APA, 2007), and institutional requirements. Such laws, guidelines, and requirements describe how long records should be maintained, the format in which they are maintained, and under which circumstances they should be released. In clinical contexts, competent adults make the decisions about who will receive copies of their reports. Patient confidentiality and care are primary considerations in the maintenance and release of records. The use and release of reports are typically discussed during the informed consent process at the outset of the assessment process.

The importance of maintaining test security and the challenges of doing so have been written about extensively (AERA, APA, & NCME, 2014; APA, 1999; Attix et al., 2007; Bush & Martin, 2006; Bush, Rapp, & Ferber, 2010; National Academy of Neuropsychology Policy and Planning Committee, 2000, 2003). The conflicting requirements between and within various ethical and legal resources can confuse clinicians and result in different approaches to managing test security. The APA (2010) Ethics Code attempts to make a distinction between test *materials* and test *data*, with different responsibilities for each (see Standards 9.04, Release of Test Data, and 9.11, Maintaining Test Security). However, for many tests this distinction is artificial, and mandates to manage them differently are impossible to satisfy: One cannot release test data and maintain security of test materials when the data are exactly the same as the test materials. For example, if a geropsychologist shows a patient a picture of a design (test material), asks the patient to copy it (test data), and the reproduction is perfect, then the test data are exactly the same as the test material. The two cannot be separated; it is impossible to release one while safeguarding the other. Geropsychologists, particularly those working in contexts in which records, including test data, are likely to be requested, need to be familiar with the issues, including various laws, explained in the relevant resources and consider how to address the situation in their practices.

Vignette

Returning to the prior case of the 92-year-old, African American woman with 7 years of education from a geographic area with known educational disparities who was administered the WAIS–IV, WMS–IV, Trail Making Test, and Wisconsin Card Sorting Test (computer version), the psychologist did not have matching norms, so it was decided to use the next closest demographically correct norms and interpret the results with caution. The patient's WAIS–IV and WMS–IV scores were corrected for age, using the 85:0 to 90:11 age range, but not for race, gender, or education; the psychologist did not have the Advanced Clinical Solutions program (NCS Pearson, 2009) or resources. Her Trail Making Test scores received full demographic corrections but only to age 85. The psychologist did not know what corrections were made for the computerized Wisconsin Card Sorting Test but had to enter her age as

90 to use the test. The patient performed very poorly on all measures, particularly those administered more than about an hour into the process. The psychologist, thinking that "interpret with caution" means avoiding making a Type II error and having the patient miss out on potentially helpful services and care, concludes that her poor performance is consistent with a diagnosis of Alzheimer's dementia and that placement in an assisted living facility or other supervised setting would be best for both the patient and her daughter. He notes that although the patient is currently independent in her home, she is likely to experience progressive functional decline in the near future. He also explains, however, that some older adults experience an immediate decline in cognitive functioning upon moving into a new residence which reflects "transfer trauma" (Hitov, 1974; Levitan, 1979), and they could have retained functioning at a higher level for a longer period of time had they remained in their own, familiar environment with appropriate supports.

Ethical Issues, Tensions, and Resources

A variety of ethical concerns are evident in this case. Questions are raised about the psychologist's competence to perform cognitive evaluations with this patient population. Although he may be competent in assessment with other patient groups or with providing other services to patients similar to the one in this case, the psychologist does not seem to have the knowledge and experience to perform a cognitive evaluation of this patient. There is no evidence that the psychologist adequately considered the patient's individual characteristics, including those associated with ethnicity, culture, or geographic norms in quality of education that, aside from cognitive ability, could affect test performance. As a result, there is a high likelihood that the services provided will either not be helpful or will result in conclusions that are harmful to the patient. In addition, the psychologist neither noted the limitations of his interpretations nor recommended additional examinations or testing by other medical providers.

The ethical conflict is between beneficence and nonmaleficence. The psychologist wants to assist the patient by contributing to the understanding of her cognitive functioning but is inadequately prepared to do so. By wanting to err on the side of maximizing safety, the recommendations may unnecessarily infringe upon her independence, which conflicts with the principle of respect for patient autonomy, thus causing considerable emotional distress. Standard 9.06, Interpreting Assessment Results, states the following:

> When interpreting assessment results, including automated interpretations, psychologists take into account the purpose of the assessment as well as the various test factors, test-taking abilities and other characteristics of the person being assessed, such as situational, personal, linguistic

and cultural differences, that might affect psychologists' judgments or reduce the accuracy of their interpretations. They indicate any significant limitations of their interpretations.

For assessments performed in forensic contexts, the *Specialty Guidelines for Forensic Psychology* (APA, 2013) offers a similar recommendation (Guideline 2.08, Appreciations of Individual and Group Differences).

The availability of tests developed and normed for persons with very advanced age and cultural diversity is quite limited, challenging any clinician faced with determining whether such cognitive loss is normal for the demographic group or reflects more pronounced pathological impairment. Even when decline is consistent with demographically similar peers, it may reflect significant loss of functions needed for managing daily affairs. When interpreting assessment results, geropsychologists must consider these issues in the context of a given patient's life and make decisions with both the patient's independence and best interests in mind. Assessment interpretations should take into account medical and neurological test results and the patient's daily requirements and available resources.

The *Standards for Educational and Psychological Testing* also states "Triangulation of multiple sources of information—including stylistic and test-taking behaviors inferred from observations during test administration—may strengthen confidence in the inference" (AERA, APA, & NCME, 2014, p. 154). Consideration of context-relevant but construct-irrelevant or construct-underrepresented behavior, such as the fatigability evidenced by the patient, is an important part of the interpretation process and one that seems to have been neglected by the psychologist. Geropsychologists consider pertinent research when making interpretations. "If the literature is incomplete, the resulting inferences may be presented with the qualification that they are hypotheses for future verification rather than probabilistic statements regarding the likelihood of some behavior that imply some known validity evidence" (AERA, APA, & NCME, 2014, p. 155).

Serial cognitive assessments can contribute confidence to the initial hypotheses. APA (2012a) Guideline 11 (Psychologists Make Appropriate Use of Longitudinal Data) describes how periodic assessments can help determine the extent and rate of cognitive change, noting that practice effects may need to be taken into account in the interpretation of subsequent test results. In addition, mean scores for many tests decline with advancing age, but appropriate normative data for longitudinal assessments may be lacking. The *Standards for Educational and Psychological Testing* states: "When making inferences about a test-taker's past, present, and future behaviors and other characteristics from test scores, the professional should consider other available data that support or challenge the inferences" (AERA, APA, & NCME,

2014, p. 154). When such information is lacking, geropsychologists describe the limitations of their assessment, including listing other possible diagnoses and the reasons for one diagnosis and set of recommendations being offered instead of another. Despite the challenges, there is a tremendous amount of information and benefit to be gained from appropriate cognitive assessment of older adults (Woodard & Axelrod, 2012).

Preferred Course of Action

The patient in this case would have been best served if the psychologist had sought consultation from a geropsychology colleague or geriatric neuropsychologist who frequently performs neuropsychological evaluations of demographically similar patients. The psychologist should have presented the findings as, at most, tentative hypotheses to be further explored with multidisciplinary exams and tests, serial cognitive and emotional assessments, and additional discussions with the patient and her daughter about the patient's functioning and safety in the home.

CONCLUSION

The psychological assessment of older adults (an integral service provided by geropsychologists) commonly serves as the foundation for psychological treatment and informs other health care providers and legal decision makers. Psychological assessment is a process that often includes, but is much broader than, psychometric testing. Each step in the assessment process, guided by ethical principles and standards, provides an opportunity to gather information that can lead to a better understanding of the patient. However, opportunities for the emergence of ethical challenges also accompany each step in the assessment process. Familiarity with relevant professional resources, practicing within the limits of professional competence, and knowing when to refer to colleagues are among the important components of ethical assessment of older adults.

5

INTERVENTION IN GEROPSYCHOLOGY

Happiness cannot be attained by wanting to be happy—it must come as the unintended consequence of working for a goal greater than oneself.
—Victor Frankl, *Man's Search for Meaning*

The overarching goal of geropsychology is "to apply scientific findings about psychological aging to improve the lives of older adults" (Qualls, 2011, p. 16). Thus, geropsychologists strive to promote the understanding and well-being of older adult patients and those involved in their lives. This goal is conceptualized broadly, and its pursuit takes many forms and occurs in a variety of settings and contexts. Such clinical services range from promoting psychological and physical well-being in healthy older adults to addressing end-of-life issues. The nature of the psychological treatment varies considerably according to individual differences in aspects of maturity, physical and psychosocial difficulties, cohort, clinical setting, and the extent to which others are involved in the patient's life (Knight, 2004). In the provision of clinical services, geropsychologists draw knowledge and skills from related psychological specialties, such as clinical and counseling psychology, health psychology, rehabilitation psychology, neuropsychology, and end-of-life care (Qualls, 2011). Such differences in patient issues, clinical contexts, and services

http://dx.doi.org/10.1037/0000010-006
Ethical Practice in Geropsychology, by S. S. Bush, R. S. Allen, and V. A. Molinari

provided correspond to differences in professional and ethical issues and challenges (Hays, 1999). Understanding the ethical issues prepares geropsychologists to provide effective clinical services.

CLARIFICATION OF CLINICAL ISSUES

Overview

Older adults receive psychological services to address a variety of problems and needs. As a group, they experience the full range of personality traits and psychological disorders, as well as more frequent sensory, motor, and medical problems and distinct lifespan development issues (Elder, 1985, 1998; Elder, Johnson, & Crosnoe, 2003). An important early step in the care of older adults is determining which issues are most troubling to the patient and hence should be the targets of initial treatment. Effective geropsychologists take care not to make assumptions based on their own biases about what a patient needs. On the basis of experience and an understanding of lifespan development literature, geropsychologists may hypothesize about the psychological needs of a patient, but they strive to understand each patient's values and the current psychological needs generated by the values. Additionally, geropsychologists understand that psychological needs can change quickly and are flexible in their approach to patient care, adapting to evolving patient needs. Clinical issues also should be distinguished from ethical, legal, or other professional issues. Despite considerable overlap, some challenges that appear to be clinical in nature may be more accurately understood as ethical dilemmas, and vice versa. Parsing out the clinical, ethical, legal, and professional components of challenging situations helps establish appropriate courses of action.

Vignette

An older adult with a recently diagnosed terminal illness has just been admitted to a long-term care facility, requiring him to leave his family and his job caring for dogs in a kennel. The psychologist consulting in the facility believes that addressing end-of-life issues or adjustment concerns related to the transition to the long-term care facility or performing a life review may be the most beneficial use of therapy sessions for the patient. The patient, however, prefers to focus on his concerns about the well-being of the dogs that he can no longer care for and the loss of his relationships with the dogs. The psychologist believes that the patient is in denial about his illness and is minimizing problems with adjustment to the long-term care facility, so she repeatedly attempts to steer discussions in those directions, which becomes such a source of frustration for the patient that he quickly begins refusing to meet with the psychologist.

Ethical Decision-Making Process

As illustrated in Exhibits 3.1 and 3.2, a sequence of ethical decision-making questions and steps provides a structured approach to addressing ethical challenges. Asking oneself the questions and following the steps for each case is likely to help achieve good outcomes. When a working knowledge of the questions and steps has been achieved, ethical challenges can often be addressed implicitly under conceptually integrated headings.

Ethical Issues, Tensions, and Resources

Efforts to provide helpful psychological services (beneficence) begin with listening to and understanding patients' concerns. Discounting patients' presenting concerns, even when more significant psychosocial issues seem readily apparent to the clinician, can have a fatal impact on rapport, causing patients to reject psychological services that could help address a variety of issues. Valuing patients' presenting concerns is consistent with the principle of respect for patient autonomy. During the informed consent process at the outset of therapy, psychologists discuss with patients the nature of therapy (Standard 10.01, Informed Consent to Therapy), which includes the goals that therapy will target. One of the most important factors for successful psychotherapy is a good therapeutic relationship, which often reflects concordance between patient and therapist goals (Ardito & Rabellino, 2011). When it becomes apparent that the patient and therapist have different goals, it is the therapist's responsibility to discuss the issue with the patient and strive to resolve it in a manner that is acceptable to both parties and beneficial to the patient.

The primary ethical tension is between beneficence as conceptualized by the psychologist and respect for patient autonomy. The psychologist and patient have different ideas about what is best for the patient, but rather than respecting his wishes or at least discussing the options with him and processing his thoughts and feelings about the options, the psychologist pushed her own agenda. General bioethical principles (Beauchamp & Childress, 2013), the *Ethical Principles of Psychologists and Code of Conduct* (American Psychological Association [APA], 2010; hereinafter, Ethics Code), and authoritative texts on psychotherapy with older adults (e.g., Knight, 2004) and interventions with individuals near the end of life (e.g., Allen et al., 2014; Chochinov, 2012; Werth & Blevins, 2006) are informative in this case.

The patient would have been best served if the psychologist had agreed to focus on the patient's concerns about the dogs and the loss of his relationships with the dogs—in other words, if the psychologist had respected the patient's choice of topics for the initial focus of therapy while maintaining an appreciation of the variety of issues that could be targets for psychological intervention. Individuals experience a variety of losses near the end of life, and this experience might have been the patient's segue into discussion of other grief issues. Addressing the loss of the dogs at the outset would have helped establish rapport and opened the door to discussion of the other issues that the psychologist identified as important and that the patient would likely also identify as important when the time was right. At this point, given the current poor rapport, the geropsychologist should either change course immediately and listen to the patient's desires or refer to another qualified professional who may be better able to set the therapy on its proper course.

WORK WITHIN ORGANIZATIONS AND TEAMS

The settings and contexts in which older adults receive psychological services overlap considerably with younger patient populations, but readily apparent differences also exist. Because of the increased health problems and unique stressors associated with aging, older adults more frequently receive psychological services in medical settings. In addition, because of medical necessity and the decreased autonomy that results from the cognitive and physical decline associated with aging, older adults are commonly treated in nontraditional settings such as adult day service programs, long-term care facilities, and their own homes. Geropsychologists working in such contexts are often part of treatment teams or, in their roles as consultants, interact closely with care providers in other specialties (O'Shea Carney, Gum, & Zeiss, 2015). Such interdisciplinary collaboration promotes patient care and well-being but can also underlie or contribute to ethical challenges (see Chapter 3).

Compared with independent practice contexts, geropsychologists working within or for organizations often interact with and receive input from administrators who, despite a shared goal of promoting patient welfare, may have different ideas about the best ways to achieve the goal or may seem to have additional goals (e.g., financial) that supersede pursuit of patient welfare. Open communication between geropsychologists and administrators in a context that values the benefits that psychological services offer to patients, their families, staff, and the overall setting can provide a rewarding professional experience. Yet, even in such ideal situations, ethical challenges arise. When the relationship between geropsychologist and administrator is less ideal, the ethical challenges and the hurdles to address them effectively are undoubtedly greater.

Older adult patients also transition between different types of care or residential settings based on medical status changes and the level of care or assistance required to meet their changing needs. Geropsychologists have a responsibility to try to facilitate transfer of psychological services when they are no longer able to continue providing treatment. Standard 10.09, Interruption of Therapy, requires psychologists to "make reasonable efforts to provide for orderly and appropriate resolution of responsibility for client/patient care" when there are changes in the psychologist's employment or contractual obligations. This approach to managing transitions in care is equally applicable when prolonged changes in a patient's level of care necessitate a change in clinicians.

Family members and close friends often play invaluable roles in the care and psychological well-being of adults in various treatment settings. Family members often bring to the patient's care an understanding of the patient that even the best-intentioned health care provider cannot. Some family members and friends also fill gaps in supervision and care that even facilities with devoted staff simply cannot always provide. However, some family members and friends, often with the patient's best interests in mind but sometimes with their own agendas or reflecting their own personality traits, can be difficult, demanding, and a source of friction and conflict with staff. While clinically taxing, the actions of some family members and friends can also lead to ethical challenges. Awareness of the potential for such challenges prepares geropsychologists to anticipate and avoid or successfully address them when they occur.

Striving to understand the values of both patients and their family members can help geropsychologists make clinical and ethical decisions that promote patients' best interests. Although patients and their family members commonly have shared values, such values may also differ in important ways that can affect patient autonomy, care, and treatment. This issue is particularly important in situations in which patients have diminished decision-making capacity. As noted in Chapter 4, performing a values assessment can help clarify similarities and differences in aspects of life and care that patients and family members consider important. Values history worksheets can facilitate this process. Such worksheets for patients are available online, and Bush (2009) provided a similar values worksheet to be used with family members.

The importance of a team approach (which includes the patient and involved family members) to the care of older adults is well understood by geropsychologists. The Pikes Peak model includes working within teams and understanding the impact of various settings on older adults among the competencies required of geropsychologists (Knight, Karel, Hinrichsen,

Qualls, & Duffy, 2009): "Several themes run throughout the model . . . The model strongly emphasizes recognizing and countering one's own explicit or implicit ageism. Interdisciplinary collaboration and the influence of a range of social environments on older adults are also emphasized" (p. 210). The APA Presidential Task Force on Integrated Health Care for an Aging Population (2008) presented a model for integrated, interdisciplinary care. Included among the model's eight basic principles is an understanding that conflicts among team members are natural and can have positive or negative effects, with psychologists serving an important function by applying conflict resolution skills to team conflicts. As Emery (2011) noted, "any setting in which older adults are receiving health care could be improved by maximizing the integration of health care providers, patients, family members, and other community members and agencies" (p. 85).

However, such integration is not without its ethical implications. For example, a primary ethical challenge in institutional and interdisciplinary settings involves privacy and confidentiality in the context of therapeutic interventions and the need to share information among team members. Compared with outpatient and independent practice settings, geropsychologists often struggle with (a) the limits on privacy inherent as a result of the physical setting, including the presence of roommates and interruptions by other staff members; and (b) the nature and amount of information about the patient's therapy to express verbally to team members and in documentation. Respecting a competent patient's autonomy and right to privacy by informing the patient about (a) known or potential intrusions on privacy, (b) anticipated limits to confidentiality, and (c) the importance for the patient's care of sharing information among team members and providing options and choices about such matters is consistent with ethical practice. Geropsychologists who are aware of both the ethical challenges and the benefits associated with interdisciplinary integration are well-positioned to provide effective services and important contributions to all parties.

Vignette

A 74-year-old man who was born and raised in an Eastern European country came to the United States as a young adult and worked in construction, barely making enough money to support his family's most basic needs. He was admitted to a hospital for acute care following a large left hemisphere stroke that left him with expressive aphasia and hemiparesis. The patient would become quite agitated at times, and so the team psychologist was asked to evaluate him. Although the patient seemed to understand basic questions and instructions, he could not respond verbally or in writing. A speech-language pathologist, who was originally from a different Eastern European country, had previously evaluated the patient using a communication board and determined that he was probably of very limited intellect prior to the stroke, definitely lacked cognitive capacity at this time to make decisions regarding his health care and discharge, and was probably prone to agitation and aggression throughout his life. That opinion was inconsistent with the psychologist's initial impression of the patient. The psychologist met with the patient's wife and again interviewed the patient using a yes–no response format. The psychologist learned that there was a history of animosity between some groups from the two Eastern European countries and that the patient's agitation seemed to occur when interacting with three staff members, including the speech therapist, who were from the other country. The patient's wife, fearing that the staff members would treat the patient poorly, asked the psychologist not to discuss these concerns with other staff members. The psychologist informed the patient and his wife that he must discuss the issue with the other team members and would do so in a sensitive fashion to improve rather than derail care. He then brought the issue to the speech therapist, who acknowledged the history of animosity but maintained that she did not let it affect her actions or opinions and did not believe it had anything to do with the patient's agitation. She refused to transfer the patient's care to another speech therapist. Later that day the attending physician, who was also the team leader, spoke to the psychologist and stated, "I understand that you've been blaming the speech therapist for the patient's agitation and low cognitive functioning. I think you're probably off target a bit here. It's best if we each do our own job in this case."

Ethical Issues, Tensions, and Resources

The psychologist's efforts to understand the patient's behavior and cognitive abilities are consistent with a desire to promote patient care (beneficence). The apparent cultural mismatch between the patient and some of the treatment team members could prove harmful to the patient's care and progress, and the psychologist attempted to reduce the potential for such harmful effects (nonmaleficence). However, in contrast to some other clinical contexts, the psychologist operates in a team context, is not the final decision maker regarding team member participation, and must work within the system to advocate for what he believes is needed to promote the patient's care. The psychologist also needs to consider the patient's wife's request when she, speaking for her husband, asked the psychologist not to share their concerns with the other team members (respect for patient autonomy).

Tensions exist between the treatment team's goal of helping the patient and the discordant cultural history between the patient and some staff members, which might have an unintended impact on assessments of the patient's psychological state, behavior, and apparent cognitive functioning. For the geropsychologist, tensions exist between the need (a) to advocate for the patient and (b) to work within the team to attempt to provide integrated care, and between the need (a) to advocate for the patient and (b) to respect the patient's wife's request for confidentiality on this matter. Standard 3.09, Cooperation With Other Professionals, states, "When indicated and professionally appropriate, psychologists cooperate with other professionals in order to serve their clients/patients effectively and appropriately." Standard 3.11, Psychological Services Delivered to or Through Organizations, states in part,

> (a) Psychologists delivering services to or through organizations provide information beforehand to clients and when appropriate those directly affected by the services about . . . (5) the probable uses of services provided and information obtained, (6) who will have access to the information, and (7) limits of confidentiality.

Standards in the Ethics Code (Standard 4, Privacy and Confidentiality; Standard 10.01, Informed Consent to Therapy) also address the need to maintain confidentiality and to inform all parties about the limits of confidentiality as early as possible in the relationship, "recognizing that the extent and limits of confidentiality may be regulated by law or established by institutional rules or professional or scientific relationship" (Standard 4.01, Maintaining Confidentiality). Consultation with a colleague who is very familiar with the Eastern European countries in question could also provide valuable insight into the cultural, interpersonal, and intrapsychic dynamics at play.

Geropsychologists do not rely on ethics resources only for their help in avoiding discrimination based on individual and cultural differences; they also value the emphasis those resources place on striving to understand how sociocultural factors (e.g., historical time and place) influence the experience and expression of health and mental health problems throughout the aging process (e.g., Administration on Aging, 2001; APA, 2004 [especially Principle 5]; APA Committee on Aging, 2009; Elder, 1985, 1998). The problem in this case is not that the patient is being discriminated against; rather, there is a lack of sensitivity by some team members to the patient's cultural experience, particularly considered within the context of the time in history in which the patient resided in his native country. In fact, the team member who may be assumed to be the most sensitive to the patient's cultural experience is actually the person who is most dismissive of cultural considerations because of differences in sociocultural history. Consistent with the concept of gerodiversity (i.e., the significant variation in older adults across a variety of demographic and psychological characteristics), cultural heritage is an important factor to consider when working with older adults (Iwasaki, Tazeau, Kimmel, Baker, & McCallum, 2009; Tazeau, 2011). In the context of multicultural consultation to organizations, social justice is a primary ethical principle because it involves removing barriers to equal access to, and opportunity for, quality care (Sue, 2008; Tazeau, 2011).

Preferred Course of Action

From the beginning of his interactions with the patient and his wife, the psychologist should have made it clear that he works as part of a team and that information discussed may be shared with the team in order to promote the patient's care. Although confidentiality between patient and psychologist is, with few exceptions, essential for psychotherapy (because it allows patients to speak freely about very personal matters), clinicians working with integrated teams have responsibilities to both the patients (including family members) and the team. The geropsychologist should have discussed with the patient and his wife the importance of sharing the cultural heritage issues with the team, underscoring the importance for the patient's care and addressing their concerns. To address the cultural issue with team members was the appropriate next step. Whether to address it first with the speech therapist or with the team leader or in a team meeting could be extensively debated. The goals would be to educate the involved parties about the apparent impact of cultural issues on the patient's periodic agitation and the possibly incorrect attributions of cognitive impairment, as well as the need to serve the patient's best interests by minimizing or eliminating contact with care providers from the Eastern European country in question. If such contact could not be avoided, then the importance of sensitivity to the patient's cultural heritage should be discussed with all team members and care providers, including the patient and his wife. If reducing or eliminating such contact was possible but cooperation from those involved was not forthcoming, the geropsychologist would need to address the matter with the next person in the decision-making hierarchy, such as an administrator, to work toward removing the barriers to quality care.

MISTREATMENT OF OLDER ADULTS

Overview

Geropsychologists at times encounter situations in which their patients are abused, neglected, or exploited. Such mistreatment takes many forms, including physical, sexual, and emotional abuse; financial or material exploitation; neglect; abandonment; and self-neglect (National Center on Elder Abuse, 1999). Reported cases of elder mistreatment have increased substantially in recent years, although the reported cases are considered a significant underestimation of the true number of cases of mistreatment (National Center on Elder Abuse, 2005). Severity of mistreatment ranges from very mild to something as extreme as death. Most abuse is perpetrated by adult children and other family members of the older adults, but abuse within institutions is becoming a growing problem as lifespan increases and more people are spending more time in medical, assisted living, and skilled nursing care settings.

Older adults, like all people, deserve to live in safety and with dignity. The Older Americans Act of 1965 was established in part to promote the peace and dignity of older adults by protecting them from mistreatment and by implementing interventions when mistreatment occurs. (The act has been amended every few years since 1965; examples include the Older Americans Act Amendments of 2006 and the Older Americans Reauthorization Technical Corrections Act of 2007.) From an ethical perspective, the APA (2010) Ethics Code, in the first line of the first principle (Principle A: Beneficence and Nonmaleficence), states, "Psychologists strive to benefit those with whom they work. . . ." Thus, in addition to legal requirements in many jurisdictions, there exists an ethical foundation for psychologists to promote the welfare of abused, neglected, or exploited older adult patients. The specific steps that geropsychologists take when confronted with evidence of mistreatment of their patients varies according to state law, with state agencies offering adult protective services. Not all states mandate reporting of elder abuse by psychologists, and in some instances doing so may violate confidentiality; nevertheless, other guidelines or terminology, such as protection of vulnerable populations, might permit or require psychologists to report mistreatment of older adult patients. Although care must be taken to respect confidentiality rights, clinicians can often take a variety of steps to protect older adult patients that do not violate confidentiality, even in the absence of a legal mandate to report the maltreatment. A multidisciplinary response to the mistreatment of older adults is now considered best practice (Brandl et al., 2007).

Vignette

An 84-year-old woman is brought to a mental health clinic for treatment of depression. During the initial interview, the patient reveals that her daughter frequently demands money from her. Although she has barely enough funds to cover her basic needs, she must give the money to her daughter or her daughter will hurt her. However, her daughter does not cause the injuries directly; rather, she hides the patient's eyeglasses so that the patient trips over or bumps into objects and falls, or her daughter will leave a puddle of water on the tile kitchen floor so that the patient slips and falls, or she will do something else that is similarly devious. The geropsychologist wonders whether the patient is inappropriately attributing her falls and injuries to nefarious actions on the part of her daughter or whether the daughter is actually doing such things. The patient strongly opposes the geropsychologist having contact with her daughter because of fear that her daughter will retaliate. The geropsychologist then informs the patient that he must make a formal report to Adult Protective Services, which the patient again opposes for the same reason. The geropsychologist reminds the patient that, as he explained during the informed consent process, he must report when there is evidence of danger to oneself, others, or older adults. The patient clarifies that she thought the geropsychologist meant that he would report if *she* were to harm an older adult. She states that she never would have agreed to those conditions or confided in him if she had known that he would report it. She then states that she will kill herself if he discusses the matter with anyone.

Ethical Issues, Tensions, and Resources

Needing to help and protect the patient is consistent with the principle of beneficence, while needing to comply with her request for privacy and confidentiality reflects respect for patient autonomy. There is also a legal mandate to report suspected elder abuse and the intention to commit suicide. A conflict exists between needing to help and protect the patient (beneficence) and needing to comply with her request for privacy and confidentiality (respect for patient autonomy). There is also a conflict between respect for patient autonomy and the legal mandate to report suspected elder abuse. State laws that protect patients typically trump aspirational ethical principles in such decisions. In this case, the patient's statement that she would kill herself could trigger additional mandated reporting requirements that result in the patient being involuntarily hospitalized. Any violation of confidentiality will have a significant adverse effect on her emotional state, her confidence in mental health care, her relationship with her daughter, and possibly her well-being. The geropsychologist also considers that the manner in which he explained the limits to confidentiality may have been inadequate, leaving him at least partially responsible for the challenge he now is facing and the distress the patient is experiencing.

Relevant resources include the Ethics Code, with a focus on Principles A (Beneficence and Nonmaleficence) and E (Respect for People's Rights and Dignity) and the Standards involving privacy and confidentiality (Standard 4) and informed consent (Standards 3.10 and 10.01, Terminating Therapy). State laws involving mandated reporting are also essential. The perspective of an experienced and trusted colleague is valuable. Scholarly works such as Brandl et al. (2007) offer direction in such challenging circumstances.

Preferred Course of Action

Needing time to think and decide what to do, the geropsychologist suggests that they take a brief break, remaining in the office, and she agrees. Next, he contacts a trusted geropsychology colleague and asks for advice about handling this complex interplay of ethical, legal, and clinical issues. The colleague recommends contacting Adult Protective Services, the ethics committee of the state psychological association, and his professional liability insurance carrier to explain the situation (without providing identifying patient information) and to seek their input. Her recommended first course of action, however, is to continue to process the issue with the patient, attempting to strike an agreement that, because she does not appear to be in imminent danger, he will not contact her daughter or Adult Protective Services at this point if she will agree not to harm herself. Although generally skeptical of the value of such "contracts" with patients, the geropsychologist does not believe the patient will have reason to harm herself if he maintains confidentiality, and she clearly states as much. The colleague also suggests asking the patient if she could stay temporarily with another family member. The geropsychologist and patient agree to a follow-up session in 2 days to continue addressing the patient's depression. The geropsychologist informs the patient that if she does not come for the follow-up appointment, he will have no choice but to make the calls necessary to determine and assure her safety, which the patient understands and to which she agrees. This plan provides the geropsychologist with the time needed to review the relevant documents and make the contacts needed to determine the best course of action.

SELECTION AND USE OF TREATMENTS

Overview

Selecting the treatment modality is an important part of the therapeutic process and is typically influenced by (a) the patient's presenting problems, in the context of his or her cognitive, emotional, and interpersonal abilities and weaknesses; (b) the treatment setting; and (c) the education, training, and experience of the therapist. Interventions such as life review therapy (e.g., Butler, 1963; Haber, 2006) that have been developed for use with older adults are appropriate for some patients, whereas the use or adaptation of psychotherapeutic modalities that are commonly used with younger populations may be preferred for other older adult patients. As Hinrichsen (2011) noted, "many psychotherapies that were originally developed for younger populations are effective for older people" (p. 58). The Pikes Peak model encourages geropsychologists to "apply individual, group, and family interventions to older adults using appropriate modifications to accommodate distinctive biopsychosocial functioning of older adults and distinct therapeutic relationship characteristics" (Knight et al., 2009, p. 213). As Qualls (2011) explained, geropsychologists commonly conceptualize patient issues and provide services within a biopsychosocial framework, considering each of these aspects of the patient's life separately and in their often complex interactions. Additionally, some interventions provided to, or for, older adults are not psychotherapy per se. For example, behavioral intervention consultation with treatment teams and education of caregivers are valuable nonpsychotherapeutic services that geropsychologists provide.

As with other patient populations, psychologists treating older adults should be familiar with the evidence base (or lack thereof) supporting their interventions. Although much of the research on evidence-based psychotherapies with older adults has involved cognitive–behavioral therapy (Gatz, 2007; Scogin & Presnell, 2011), empirical support for a variety of other interventions also exists for use with, or on behalf of, older adults (Scogin, Welsh, Hanson, Stump, & Coates, 2005). No single psychotherapeutic modality has emerged as preferable with older adults (APA, 2004, Guideline 14). Despite a considerable and growing evidence base supporting various interventions with older adults, there remain gaps in the literature that geropsychologists should be aware of when selecting treatment modalities (see Gatz, 2007, for an overview).

Applying psychological principles and techniques to improving the lives of older adults is not limited to addressing diseases, disorders, or disabilities. A substantial portion of the general population goes to great lengths to live healthier longer, and cognitive and emotional health is no exception. Although some early efforts to satisfy the hopes of consumers seemed more like snake oil than science, there is now a growing evidence base to support efforts to maximize brain wellness. For example, research shows the neurocognitive benefits of a variety of biopsychosocial interventions (e.g., Ball et al., 2002; Carlson, 2011; James, Wilson, Barnes, & Bennett, 2011; McDougall et al., 2010; Richmond, Morrison, Chein, & Olson, 2011; Willis et al., 2006; Wilson et al., 2002). Experience indicates that older adults are increasingly turning to websites that purport to offer brain wellness and memory promotion activities, some for a fee, commonly asking geropsychologists whether it is "worth it." Some product marketing campaigns and media presentations, perhaps preying upon older adults' fears of getting a progressive dementia, may offer a more promising picture of the benefits of their products than science supports. Unfortunately, older adults and their families may accept these advertisements and promotional materials based on their hope that the product or service will work for them rather than reviewing the materials with a reasonable degree of skepticism. Geropsychologists can provide a valuable service by critically reviewing the "science" that reportedly supports health promotion products or services and by summarizing the information for their clients, fostering reasonable expectations. There appears to be great potential for geropsychologists to serve older adults in this new and exciting aspect of professional service as long as realistic, evidence-based expectations are established.

Understanding when to end treatment is as important as deciding whether to start treatment or which treatment modality to use. According to the Ethics Code (Standard 10.10, Terminating Therapy), psychologists should "terminate therapy when it becomes reasonably clear that the client/patient no longer needs the service, is not likely to benefit, or is being harmed by continued service." However, *need* and *benefit* can be challenging concepts to operationally define with some older adult populations and in some clinical contexts. Quantitative outcome measures may not reflect the benefits of treatment, particularly when treatment helps to maintain a given level of functioning that would otherwise deteriorate faster. Geropsychologists have much to offer beyond traditional psychotherapy with relatively high-functioning patients but must be cautious when considering providing and billing for services that may be just as effectively provided by an untrained volunteer; there could be ethical and legal ramifications.

The Office of the Inspector General, through its Office of Evaluation and Inspections, determined that 27% of psychiatric services provided in nursing homes are medically unnecessary, with Medicare payments for such services being inappropriate:

> More than half of unnecessary services are provided to individuals whose cognitive limitations make them unable to benefit from the psychiatric intervention, and about half have an inappropriate frequency and/or duration. Additionally, many medically unnecessary services do not appear to stabilize or improve patients' conditions. (U.S. Department of Health and Human Services, Office of the Inspector General, 2001, p. ii)

The Office of the Inspector General also determined that psychological testing was the most problematic mental health service that was reviewed; 39% of the psychological tests that were administered were medically unnecessary because they are too long, too frequent, or not needed by the patient. Some of the problems identified by the Office of the Inspector General dealt with clinicians' lack of adequate documentation even though appropriate services were actually delivered and local carriers not properly defining procedures for coding testing. Thus, when offering necessary and beneficial services, particularly to patient groups such as those described by the Office of the Inspector General, geropsychologists are well-served by clearly documenting the rationale, and the evidence, supporting their services.

Most recently, the U.S. Department of Justice completed its "largest criminal health care fraud takedown in the history of the Department of Justice," resulting in charges against 243 individuals for approximately $712 million in false Medicare billing. Among those charged were mental health professionals who billed for psychotherapy and other services that were considered by investigators to have been unnecessary.

> In one case, administrators in a mental health center billed close to $64 million between 2006 and 2012 for purported intensive mental health treatment to beneficiaries and allegedly paid kickbacks to patient recruiters and assisted living facility owners throughout the Southern District of Florida. (U.S. Department of Justice, Office of Public Affairs, 2015)

Geropsychologists who are committed to high standards of ethical and legal practice and want to avoid being lumped in with those who are intentionally engaging in fraud must be very careful to provide evidence-based services that are psychologically necessary and to accurately and thoroughly document the necessity for and nature of the services.

Vignette

A geropsychologist attends a workshop that presents exciting research on the potential cognitive exercise has to improve memory functioning in healthy older adults. She sees in this research an opportunity to help a lot of older adults and generate a new and lucrative revenue stream. Upon returning to her office, she reviews research on the topic, which reveals that in some studies intensive attention training helped to enhance certain types of cognitive abilities in the short term, but other studies did not find this effect. To improve on these findings, she purchases some computer-based attention tasks that she is familiar with and loads them into five laptops. She then creates a brochure describing her service to prevent Alzheimer's disease and quoting selectively from the research studies. She begins promoting her new service to the community. She also takes the laptops with her twice a week when she consults in an assisted living facility, where she sets up five residents on the laptops at the same time. She then writes her progress notes while the computerized attention programs run. After 30 minutes, she does the same thing with another five residents. She bills Medicare for the "treatment," which was not at all similar to the procedures used in the studies that she had read.

Ethical Issues, Tensions, and Resources

Presenting attention exercises as a guaranteed prevention for Alzheimer's disease is grossly misleading, establishes unrealistic expectations, and can contribute to frustration and sadness for patients and their families if a neuro-cognitive disorder is later diagnosed. Thus, the service is very unlikely to be helpful and could reasonably be expected to result in psychological harm at some point in the future. Ethical principles of beneficence, nonmaleficence, justice, integrity, and respect for autonomy are all relevant.

There is a conflict between the geropsychologist's genuine wish to help older adults (beneficence) and her use of unsubstantiated methods and proce-dures, possibly driven in part by greed, to accomplish her goal. She wants to capture the exciting and promising work being conducted by researchers and to apply it in the real world, but her approach is misguided. Her methods and procedures, promoted by exaggerated claims of benefit, are very unlikely to be helpful and could have harmful consequences (nonmaleficence). Failing to present the service in a more balanced manner that allows patients to make a more truly informed decision about participation is unfair and inconsistent with respect for patient autonomy. Indeed, questionable billing practices may be fraudulent and have legal consequences.

Principle C (Integrity) states: "Psychologists seek to promote accuracy, honesty, and truthfulness in the science, teaching, and practice of psychology. In these activities psychologists do not steal, cheat, or engage in fraud, sub-terfuge, or intentional misrepresentation of fact." Principle D (Justice) states: "Psychologists exercise reasonable judgment and take precautions to ensure that their potential biases, the boundaries of their competence and the limitations of their expertise do not lead to or condone unjust practices." Standard 2.04, Bases for Scientific and Professional Judgments, states: "Psychologists' work is based upon established scientific and professional knowledge of the discipline." Standard 10.01, Informed Consent to Therapy, states,

> (b) When obtaining informed consent for treatment for which generally recognized techniques and procedures have not been established, psy-chologists inform their clients/patients of the developing nature of the treatment, the potential risks involved, alternative treatments that may be available and the voluntary nature of their participation.

Standard 5.01, Avoidance of False or Deceptive Statements, section (b) states, in part, that psychologists do not make false, deceptive, or fraudulent state-ments concerning their services, or about the scientific or clinical basis for, or results or degree of success of, their services.

The APA Presidential Task Force on Evidence-Based Practice (2006) described evidence-based practice as being composed of three elements: use of the best available scientific information, clinician expertise, and client val-ues and preferences. Although the geropsychologist described in the vignette was informed by solid (albeit selective) scientific information, she diverged so wildly from the procedures used in the studies as to render any comparison meaningless. Additionally, she had no prior expertise in this aspect of practice, and, by failing to provide information needed for truly informed consent, she did not adequately consider her patients' values and preferences. Thus, her "treatments" were not consistent with evidence-based practice and raise concerns about professional competence.

Preferred Course of Action

Managing patient expectations, which requires sharing with them complete and accurate information about the proposed services, is a primary goal when using developing or alternative treatments. The geropsychologist had a responsibility to inform her patients that, although informed by theory and science, there was essentially no empirical base for her proposed treatment. As a result, the potential benefits are unknown, but the potential risks appear to be few. Her billing decisions should also be reconsidered.

CULTURE AND COHORT ISSUES

Overview

Individual and cohort differences in the psychological treatment of older adults bring richness to the process that adds value to the professional experience but can also pose clinical and ethical challenges. Cultural, racial, gender, sexual orientation, cohort, and other differences may exist between patients and clinicians, between patients and other health care providers, between patients and their family members, and between the geriatric patients treated in the same clinical setting. Such differences may affect selection and application of assessment measures and normative data, choice of treatment method, and involvement of persons other than the patient and clinician in the evaluation or treatment. Individual or cohort differences may even affect the patient's willingness to participate in psychological services or interact with a specific clinician at all. Sensitivity to individual and cohort differences and a genuine desire to understand each patient's perspective about such differences maximizes the potential for older adults to receive good clinical care. There are more similarities than differences among most people, and it is the similarities, in the context of a desire to understand the influences of the differences, that serve as the foundation for mutual understanding and beneficial clinical care. Actual or perceived lack of such sensitivity to differences allows little opportunity for the provision of culturally competent care with older adult populations.

Vignette

A geropsychologist working in a long-term care facility in a large urban setting believes that patients on the palliative care unit would benefit from group therapy to examine and process their thoughts and feelings about end-of-life issues with others who are going through similar experiences. While respectful of the rights of patients to decline services, the geropsychologist never considers that these patients, some of whom she treats in individual psychotherapy, would not want to participate in the group. She takes a rather paternalistic and direct approach to getting group participants for the initial session, telling them that they should trust her that this activity will have positive effects for them. The group's eight initial participants consist of men and women (a) of four different races, representing a couple of different cultural groups within the same racial groups; (b) in different socioeconomic classes; (c) who have five different religious affiliations; (d) with eight different medical problems and types of disability; and (e) who range in age from 63 to 92 years. After orienting everyone to the group's nature and purpose, the geropsychologist is surprised that the group members are silent. With considerable prompting, one member of the group begins talking and becomes reluctant to stop, even with prompting from the geropsychologist when another group member appears to have a comment. The geropsychologist is disappointed to learn the following week that only two members of the group were willing to return, one of whom was the person who monopolized the conversation. Also, two of the group members who participated in individual psychotherapy with the geropsychologist terminated their individual therapy, with little explanation.

Ethical Issues, Tensions, and Resources

The desire to provide a potentially valuable service (beneficence) to a group of patients dealing with end-of-life challenges and opportunities motivated the geropsychologist to form the therapy group. However, failure to perform a needs assessment to gauge interest in such a group and to consider and prepare for the diversity among the group members was a significant flaw in the planning and implementation of the group. Failure to engage each possible participant in an appropriate informed consent process was inconsistent with the respect for patient autonomy required of clinicians.

This case does not reflect tension between two competing ethical principles as much as it illustrates how one principle can be compromised in pursuit of another. Specifically, respect for patient autonomy, which includes informed consent and respect for individual differences, was compromised in the pursuit of beneficence. Familiarity with the values, beliefs, and preferences of different patient populations with whom one works promotes good practice. Principle E (Respect for People's Rights and Dignity) states,

> Psychologists are aware of and respect cultural, individual and role differences, including those based on age, gender, gender identity, race, ethnicity, culture, national origin, religion, sexual orientation, disability, language and socioeconomic status and consider these factors when working with members of such groups.

More particular to older adults, Hinrichsen (2006) explained, "For those who work with specific racial and ethnic minority aged, it is especially useful to understand the larger historical, cultural, economic, social, and political forces that may have influenced and continue to influence their clients' lives" (p. 34). This approach to geropsychological services appears to be consistent with gerodiversity (Iwasaki et al., 2009; Tazeau, 2011).

Despite familiarity with cultural norms, geropsychologists "should not assume that because a patient belongs to a particular community or culture, he or she affirms that community's worldview and values" (Beauchamp & Childress, 2013, p. 110). Aging individuals within different ethnic groups vary widely in terms of their assimilation and acculturation to the dominant culture (Jang, Kim, Chiriboga, & King-Kallimanis, 2007). For example, compared with European Americans and African Americans, Korean Americans and Mexican Americans tend to believe that the family, rather than the individual, should make decisions about the use of life support (Gert, Culver, & Clouser, 2006). Nevertheless, consistent with the principle that affirms respecting patient autonomy, persons from each ethnic group should be given the choice of whether they want to make such decisions or delegate the decisions to others. Patients have a *right* to choose, including choosing whether to accept information at all, but no *duty* to choose; clinicians, however, have a duty to present the choice, if not the information to the patient (Beauchamp & Childress, 2013).

Generational or cohort differences are underappreciated aspects of diversity. Consistent with the information presented by Hinrichsen (2006), Principle 5 of the APA (2004) *Guidelines for Psychological Practice With Older Adults* (citing Knight & Lee, 2008) informs readers that perspectives on many aspects of life differ from cohort to cohort and will continue to change over time, profoundly influencing "the experience and expression of health and psychological problems" (p. 40). This principle clearly illustrates the role of historical time and place in life course development (Elder, 1985, 1998).

Consistent with cultural competence, geropsychologists practicing in a manner consistent with the Pikes Peak model are sensitive to the complex interaction of diversity and aging. However, as with other aspects of professional competence, cultural competence is not static, and its attainment does not render geropsychologists immune to sometimes losing track of aspects of diversity and the potential impact of diversity on their decisions regarding assessment, treatment, consultation, and program development. Much is made of sensitivity to diversity and cohort issues, as it should be. Sensitivity, however, is simply the foundation; the knowledge gained from sensitivity must be translated into improved services for older adults. Similarly, openness to information about individual and group differences, often described as important, is vital but often insufficient in its passivity; it is necessary for geropsychologists to strive more actively to gain information about the potential impact of diversity and cohort differences on patients' life experiences, values, and perceptions of health, illness, coping, and care.

Preferred Course of Action

As part of her preparation, the geropsychologist should have given more thought to group composition and to the possible influence of diversity and cohort differences on group members and the success of the group. She should then have better informed potential patients of the purpose, nature, and expectations of the group, including the diverse nature of the participants; elicited and answered any questions or concerns; determined the patients' interest in participating; and sought their fully informed consent. Sensitivity to such issues and a willingness to process the issues and address challenges should also continue after the group gets underway.

PRIVACY, CONFIDENTIALITY, AND PRIVILEGE

What I may see or hear in the course of the treatment or even outside of the treatment in regard to the life of men, which on no account one must spread abroad, I will keep to myself, holding such things shameful to be spoken about.

—From the Hippocratic Oath

Overview

Western society has long considered privacy a primary value and fundamental right (Smith-Bell & Winslade, 1999), with the specific rights and restrictions having been established in the United States at both the federal and state levels. Although the word *privacy* is not found in the U.S. Constitution, the U.S. Supreme Court has recognized privacy to be a constitutional right (Eisenstadt v. Baird, 1972; Griswold v. Connecticut, 1965; Hawaii Psychiatric Society v. Ariyoshi, 1979). Despite the premium traditionally placed on privacy in health care, the protection of sensitive disclosures by patients is not absolute, and limits to privacy have been established by the courts (*Bowers v. Hardwick*, 1985; *Roe v. Wade*, 1973; *Tarasoff v. Regents of the University of California*, 1976; *Whalen v. Roe*, 1976). For example, when safety is at issue, especially for vulnerable individuals such as children, persons with disabilities, and older adults, promotion of safety outweighs the patient's right to privacy.

Privacy, confidentiality, and *privilege* are related terms involving the protection of communications from patients to clinicians in a professional context. *Privacy* is the right of individuals to determine the personal information that is shared with others. Privacy, based on the principle of respect for autonomy (Beauchamp & Childress, 2013), is a fundamental human right, reflecting freedom of self-determination and promoting dignity (Koocher & Keith-Spiegel, 1998). *Confidentiality*, based on the right to privacy, establishes limits on the release of patient information. Confidentiality can be considered a subset of privacy; as Beauchamp and Childress (2013) stated,

> The basic difference between the right to privacy and the right to confidentiality is that an infringement of a person's right to confidentiality occurs only if the person or institution to whom the information was disclosed in confidence fails to protect the information or deliberately discloses it to someone without first-party consent. By contrast, a person who, without authorization, obtains hospital records or gains access to a computer's database violates rights of privacy but does not violate rights of confidentiality. (pp. 316–317)

Privilege, a narrower concept than confidentiality, relieves the clinician from having to testify in court about a patient's communications. By "invoking privilege," the patient prevents the clinician from testifying or releasing records about intimate personal details (Behnke, Perlin, & Bernstein, 2003). By "waiving privilege," the patient allows the clinician to testify or release records in a legal proceeding. For competent adult patients, the patient is the "holder of" privilege and makes decisions about whether to invoke or waive it. Thus, while some privacy is surrendered when patients grant clinicians access to their personal information, they maintain a significant degree of control over the information (Beauchamp & Childress, 2013).

In the context of psychotherapy and related services, confidentiality serves as the foundation of trust, which is a prerequisite for many beneficial psychological services. Confident in the knowledge that their innermost thoughts and sensitive aspects of their lives can be safely shared, patients receiving psychological services benefit from open and honest communication with the clinician. Failure to honor the patient's expectation of confidentiality can (a) destroy the patient's trust in the clinician, the treatment, and the profession; (b) possibly harm the patient in significant ways; and (c) end the patient's willingness to participate in needed future treatment with any clinician. With diagnostic accuracy and the usefulness of recommendations dependent upon the accuracy and completeness of relevant patient information, the need for patient openness and honesty is as important for assessment as it is for treatment.

Vignette

An 82-year-old man residing with his wife in an assisted living facility is about to begin an initial intake interview with a geropsychologist. The interview is being held in the patient's room, with his wife present. The patient is much higher functioning than his wife, who has relatively significant sensory and neurological problems. The geropsychologist asks the patient whether the interview should be held in private, at which point the patient states, "Don't worry; she has no idea what's going on," which actually seems to be the case based on initial observations. About 10 minutes into the interview, with the geropsychologist entering the information into his laptop computer, the door opens and a woman who appears to be in her 40s enters the room. She nods to the geropsychologist and then says to the patient, "Hi, Hon, I just need the debit card." The patient points to his wallet on a table. The woman says, "Awesome, thanks, I'll be back later," kisses the patient on the forehead, and leaves. The bewildered geropsychologist asks, "Who was that?" The patient replies, "My girlfriend. I think our three-week anniversary is tomorrow." The patient's wife has been staring at the TV the entire time and did not react to the presence of the younger woman or her husband's statements.

Over the course of the interview, the geropsychologist determines that the patient has considerable anxiety and may have more problems with cognition than he initially suspected. He asks permission to update the patient's only other relative, his daughter who resides out of state. The patient refuses and states, "In fact, I don't want you telling anyone about my girlfriend." After confirming their next appointment, the geropsychologist goes to a quiet area of the facility (he does not have an office in the facility) to finish his report, which mentions the patient's girlfriend and expresses concerns about the patient's judgment. After a while he makes a quick trip to the restroom. Upon his return, he finds the patient's girlfriend reading the report on his laptop, and she is angry. She demands, "Exactly what did he tell you? If you don't tell me, I'll report that you left private patient information lying around."

Ethical Issues, Tensions, and Resources

Many ethical issues are evident in this case. Primary among the issues are (a) the geropsychologist's desire and attempt to understand the patient's psychological needs so that appropriate services can be provided (benefi-cence); (b) the geropsychologist's appreciation of the patient's desire not to have information shared with his daughter (respect for patient autonomy); (c) the need to address concerns about the patient's judgment and the pos-sibility of financial exploitation (beneficence); and (d) his own inability to maintain confidential the patient's information on his laptop, which could prove harmful to the patient (nonmaleficence) and his own career.

The primary tension is between the geropsychologist's desire to help this patient (beneficence) and the patient's reluctance to have important infor-mation shared with anyone (respect for patient autonomy). Additionally, the geropsychologist must decide whether to share additional patient informa-tion with the patient's girlfriend by breaching confidentiality and colluding with the girlfriend, by seeking the patient's permission to share the informa-tion, or risking having his apparently unethical disclosure of confidential information reported.

Many threats to confidentiality arise in the practice of geropsychology. Examples of such threats include the following: (a) practical limitations associated with inpatient and residential settings, such as roommates and staff; (b) involvement of a treatment team; (c) requests for services by third parties, such as family members, attorneys, or organizations; (d) mandated reporting requirements, such as danger to self or others, including neglect, abuse, or exploitation of older adults or vulnerable populations; (e) billing and compliance services and organizations; (f) technological breaches or mistakes; and (g) litigation (Bush, 2009). A few of these threats are present in this case.

Research has supported the long-held impression that individuals express their thoughts and feelings more freely when they believe the informa-tion will not be shared with others. There is a reduced willingness to disclose personal information when individuals are informed that there are limits to confidentiality (Haut & Muehleman, 1986; Nowell & Spruill, 1993; Woods & McNamara, 1980), especially for patients with more severe problems (Taube & Elwork, 1990). Perhaps because of a desire to facilitate patient openness or an insufficient appreciation of the importance of educating patients about the limits of confidentiality, many clinicians do not provide full disclosure of the limits of confidentiality (Baird & Rupert, 1987), which misleads patients and can adversely affect treatment.

Standard 4: Privacy and Confidentiality describes the *primary* responsi-bility of psychologists to take reasonable precautions to protect patient infor-mation. Patients are to be informed of the limits of confidentiality and the conditions under which confidential information may be disclosed as mandated (e.g., danger to self or others; abuse, neglect, or exploitation of older adults or other vulnerable populations) or permitted by law (e.g., to provide needed professional services, obtain appropriate professional consultations, protect persons from harm, or obtain payment). In most situations, it is important at the outset of the service, and thereafter as needed, to clarify with all involved parties, including organizations, the nature and extent of the information that will, and will not, be communicated among those involved (Standards 3.07, Third-Party Requests for Services; 3.11, Psychological Services Delivered to or Through Organizations; 4.02, Discussing the Limits of Confidentiality). Such communication helps to prevent misunderstandings and strong emotional reactions when the geropsychologist chooses not to share information with others about, or provided by, a patient.

HIPAA's (1996) *privacy rule* covers the privacy of health care information. State laws also address the obligations of psychologists regarding privacy and confidentiality. Geropsychologists comply with the law that affords the patient greatest privacy.

When a determination has been made that confidential information must be disclosed, it is important to establish which information will be disclosed and the manner in which the information will be conveyed. In making these determinations, it is advantageous to consider two principles: the parsimony principle and the law of no surprises (Behnke et al., 2003). According to the parsimony principle, only the information necessary to achieve the purpose of the disclosure should be released. According to the law of no surprises, all reasonable steps should be taken to inform patients at the outset of the relationship of the circumstances under which disclosure of information to a third party will occur. It is good practice to not have clients be surprised when confidential information is disclosed; disclosing confidential information is a process that should be performed together with the client whenever possible.

Interestingly, and perhaps sadly, some ethicists have argued that the traditional idea of confidentiality in medicine is a concept that is eroding because the ideal, as traditionally understood by both patients and clinicians, no longer exists (Beauchamp & Childress, 2013). These authors have noted that in health care, confidentiality rules are widely ignored and violated in practice. Because of the need for efficient access to information in medicine and for the perceived best interests of the patient, confidentiality is regularly compromised in routine clinical care. With the emergence of electronic storage and dissemination of patient information, as well as informal discussions (e.g., with spouses and friends), "confidentiality is indeed a decrepit practice in many settings and improving the security of information through technological measures will probably not be adequate to protect all of the interests traditionally protected by rules of confidentiality" (Beauchamp & Childress, 2013, p. 318). Thus, it has been argued, medical confidentiality no longer exists. Nevertheless, the patient's right still exists, and geropsychologists have a primary ethical obligation to strive to preserve confidentiality to the extent possible.

Regarding the girlfriend of the patient in this case, there is well-established history of older adults being victimized by others preying on their vulnerabilities, such as loneliness or the desire for intimacy. Commonly referred to as the "sweetheart scam," residents in long-term care settings can be particularly vulnerable to such affections.

> However, it is discriminatory to assume that the older adult, simply because of age, cannot "see through" the scam and make an informed choice about the relationship and dispersion of finances. . . . Mental health professionals must respect the autonomous decision making of competent older adults just as with younger adults. (Bush, 2009, p. 72)

In such situations, respect for patient autonomy trumps a more paternalistic approach, no matter how disappointing or frustrating it may be for the patient's family members, facility staff, or others involved in the patient's life. However, when considering the relative strength of the principle of beneficence compared with respect for patient autonomy by maintaining confidentiality, Beauchamp and Childress (2013) stated, "Even if a compelling obligation exists such as protection of confidentiality, requirements of beneficence will in some cases override it" (p. 208).

Preferred Course of Action

The geropsychologist (and thus the patient) will probably be best served by the geropsychologist seeking additional information, regarding both the patient's cognitive status and the involvement of his daughter. A neuropsychological evaluation could determine cognitive status, and discussions with staff could help clarify how involved the patient's daughter has been and the nature of their relationship. At this point in the situation, it is feasible to inform the patient's girlfriend that he plans to obtain more information before arriving at a case conceptualization and finalizing any documentation. The geropsychologist can assure her that a feedback session is typically held at the conclusion of the evaluation and that she can ask the patient if she can be present. Alternatively, the girlfriend can ask the patient what he said during the evaluation, including the intake interview that was just held, and the geropsychologist can inform her that he is bound by patient confidentiality not to discuss the case with anyone else. If the girlfriend persists with threats about reporting, the geropsychologist can encourage her to take whatever steps she deems necessary, keeping in mind that she is the one who read confidential patient information on a private computer. Of course, he assumed risk by leaving his laptop unattended and may be held accountable for that lapse in judgment.

CONCLUSION

Geropsychologists work to promote the understanding and well-being of older adult patients through many clinical avenues and in a variety of treatment contexts. The nature of the psychological treatment is based on individual characteristics related to maturity, physical and psychosocial difficulties, cohort, clinical setting, and the extent to which others are involved in the patient's life. Each of these factors provides opportunities to connect in meaningful ways with patients and their families, and each has varying ethical obligations and potential pitfalls. Obtaining and maintaining awareness and understanding of the ethical issues allows geropsychologists to provide treatment in a manner that is consistent with high standards of ethical practice, whereas failure to do so may compromise otherwise promising care.

6

CONSULTATION, ADMINISTRATION, AND BUSINESS PRACTICES IN GEROPSYCHOLOGY

Alone we can do so little; together we can do so much.
—Helen Keller

Many geropsychologists spend much or all of their time involved in activities other than direct patient care. Among their many responsibilities, geropsychologists consult with a variety of individuals and organizations, perform administrative services at various levels of institutional hierarchies, and engage in billing and other business aspects of practice. Each of these professional activities provides opportunities for geropsychologists to identify unique ethical issues, anticipate challenges, and strive to maintain high standards of ethical practice. However, failure to take these steps can adversely affect the geropsychologist's ability to provide otherwise valuable services to other professionals and organizations and to promote the well-being and interests of older adults. Skills in consultation and business aspects of practice are among the foundational competencies expected of geropsychologists, and skills in administration and management reflect advanced or leadership competencies for geropsychologists (Knight, Karel, Hinrichsen, Qualls, & Duffy, 2009).

http://dx.doi.org/10.1037/0000010-007
Ethical Practice in Geropsychology, by S. S. Bush, R. S. Allen, and V. A. Molinari

CONSULTING WITH OTHER PROFESSIONALS
AND FAMILY MEMBERS

Overview

With appropriate consent from patients or surrogate decision makers, geropsychologists promote the treatment and well-being of patients by interacting, collaborating, and consulting with others who are involved in their patients' care or personal lives. As Knight et al. (2009) noted, psychologists working with older adults should have "awareness of the broad array of potential clients (e.g., family members, other caregivers, health care professionals, and organizations) for psychological consultation and intervention and appropriate intervention strategies in these contexts" (Knowledge Base D6, p. 213). Consultation and close collaboration with other clinicians allows for an exchange of information and ideas that is consistent with a multidisciplinary, biopsychosocial approach to promoting patient care. Such consultation and collaboration are particularly important when working with older adults because the more frequent and intensive interaction of mental and physical illness caused by multiple comorbidities in this population requires involvement of more than one clinician. Additionally, with the increasing transition to integrative care models, geropsychologists in many settings work more closely than ever before with colleagues from other disciplines and, as such, will have a responsibility to communicate complex psychological conceptualizations and other information "in a concise and useful manner" (Knight et al., 2009, Skill D4, p. 214). Consistent with the model proposed by the APA Presidential Task Force on Integrated Health Care for an Aging Population (2008) and the Pikes Peak model (Knight et al., 2009), competencies expected of geropsychologists working in integrated care settings have been described (Emery, 2011; Karel, Emery, Molinari, & the CoPGTP Task Force on the Assessment of Geropsychology Competencies, 2010). The competencies, which are summarized in Exhibit 6.1, emphasize working with interprofessional teams and systems.

Family members of older adult patients provide valuable background information and personal knowledge of the patient, which can inform psychological assessments and be useful in the development of a psychological treatment or discharge plan. Family members are also excellent sources of information about patients' cultural backgrounds, values, and religious beliefs. In addition to obtaining information from family members, psychologists provide educational information to family members and other caregivers about prevention, wellness, disorders, safety considerations, and psychological services that are planned or being provided. Family members and other caregivers are essential partners in behavioral interventions, helping

EXHIBIT 6.1
Expected Competencies for Geropsychologists in Integrated Care Settings

- Able to participate in interprofessional teams, including understanding and valuing the roles and conceptual models of other disciplines and respecting team experiences and values
- Able to address complex biopsychosocial issues by collaborating with other disciplines
- Able to communicate psychological concepts and information in a useful manner
- Able to perform systems analysis and facilitate organizational change
- Able to design and participate in multiple service delivery models, including building geriatric care teams based on theory and science
- Able to collaborate and coordinate with relevant agencies

Note. Data from Knight, Karel, Hinrichsen, Qualls, and Duffy (2009); Emery (2011); and Karel, Emery, Molinari, and the CoPGTP Task Force on the Assessment of Geropsychology Competencies (2010).

to establish and reinforce behavioral modification plans and environmental changes. Geropsychologists commonly also deliver direct care to family members in the form of individual therapy, support groups, and couples and family therapy. Geropsychologists may also offer individual services to family members coping with caregiving or other issues involving older adults.

Geropsychologists interacting with other professionals and patients' family members and other caregivers have a responsibility to be aware of the ethical issues that exist and the challenges that can arise with such interactions. Standards 3.09, Cooperation with Other Professionals, and 3.11, Psychological Services Delivered to or Through Organizations, address issues arising from the frequent interprofessional collaboration and consultation in institutional settings. Principle B (Fidelity and Responsibility) states,

> Psychologists consult with, refer to, or cooperate with other professionals and institutions to the extent needed to serve the best interests of those with whom they work. They are concerned about the ethical compliance of their colleagues' scientific and professional conduct. (American Psychological Association [APA], 2010)

The involvement of persons other than the patient requires a focus on multiple general bioethical principles and specific ethical standards. The sharing of information about patients' psychological functioning has the intended purpose of promoting patient care and well-being, consistent with the principle of beneficence, and failure to do so in an appropriate manner can be harmful, which is inconsistent with the principle of nonmaleficence. Violations of patient privacy and confidentiality (Standard 4: Privacy and Confidentiality) are among the primary ethical risks when consulting with others. For competent patients, the sharing of information occurs with the patient's approval. The patient decides what information will be shared and with whom the geropsychologist can communicate, based on information conveyed by the geropsychologist about the reasons for the communication. In some contexts, patients are informed at the outset that participation in the treatment program requires communication among clinicians, and in some contexts, such as certain forensic settings, the patient's permission for information to be released to the referral source or court may not be required. Nevertheless, even when the patient's consent to release information is not required, the patient is informed of the intended recipient and uses of the information.

Because older adults commonly receive psychological services in settings in which family members may be closely involved, such as their homes or long-term care facilities, or rely on family members for assistance getting to and from appointments, geropsychologists need to carefully consider when and how to involve family members in a manner that both benefits the patient and respects the patient's autonomy. As with consultation with other professionals, interactions with family members involve consideration of beneficence and nonmaleficence, respect for patient autonomy, privacy and confidentiality, and discussion of the limits of confidentiality during the informed consent process (Standards 4.02, Discussing the Limits of Confidentiality, and 3.10, Informed Consent). Attention to these and related ethical issues and their unique applications in different evaluation and treatment venues facilitates good clinical care.

Vignette

A geropsychologist working as part of an interprofessional team organized through an outpatient primary care practice in an urban setting evaluates a 75-year-old Filipino woman who has a variety of nonspecific somatic symptoms for which other doctors have been unable to find medical causes. The patient presents with her husband. On the basis of the information obtained in the interview of the patient and her husband, the geropsychologist becomes concerned that a specific medical disorder has been overlooked. The geropsychologist is unable to connect with the busy primary care physician who examined the patient, so he speaks to the physician assistant, who, after listening to the geropsychologist's opinion, restates that there is no medical cause for the symptoms and that the problem must be psychological. The geropsychologist takes his concern to the director of the practice, who states, "I understand and appreciate your concerns, but we really need you to focus on the psychological issues." The geropsychologist states, "I'm happy to address the psychological issues, but I also believe I have an obligation to recommend that the patient get a second opinion." The director replies, "If you do that, we will no longer need your services here."

Ethical Decision-Making Process

As illustrated in Exhibits 3.1 and 3.2, a sequence of ethical decision-making questions and steps provides a structured approach to addressing ethical challenges. Asking oneself the questions and following the steps for each case is likely to help achieve good outcomes. When a working knowledge of the questions and steps has been achieved, they can often be addressed implicitly under conceptually integrated headings.

Ethical Issues, Tensions, and Resources

A variety of ethical and professional issues are relevant in this case, including Principle A (Beneficence and Nonmaleficence); Principle B (Fidelity and Responsibility); Standards 2.01, Boundaries of Competence; 3.07, Third-Party Requests for Services; 3.09, Cooperation with Other Professionals; and 3.11, Psychological Services Delivered to or Through Organizations. The geropsychologist has an obligation to assist the patient but must do so within the boundaries of his professional competence. Facilitating appropriate patient care involves collaborating and cooperating with the other health care providers in the practice.

The geropsychologist's obligation to assist the patient (beneficence), based on what he considers beneficial, has resulted in a conflict with other members of the interprofessional health care team as well as the director of the practice. The geropsychologist has possibly overstepped the bounds of his professional competence and acted in a manner that is beyond his agreed-upon role on the team, but he will lose his job if he does what he thinks is right. As a result, a tension exists between the principle of beneficence and aspects of the principle fidelity and responsibility and ethical standards that involve cooperating with other professionals and working within established professional roles.

The *Ethical Principles of Psychologists and Code of Conduct* (APA, 2010; hereinafter, Ethics Code) is the primary resource in this case. The geropsychologist also contacts the ethics committee of his state psychological association for advice, and he contacts his personal attorney to determine whether the director of the practice would have sufficient grounds to fire him if he is simply doing what he believes is in the patient's best interests.

Preferred Course of Action

The geropsychologist understands that the ethical mandate to cooperate with other professionals does not mean that psychologists must agree or cooperate with everything that other professionals say or want. Rather, there is a responsibility to challenge actions or opinions that may be detrimental to patients. He informs the patient and her husband that they may benefit from a second opinion regarding the patient's medical symptoms. He will continue to work with the patient in the context of psychological adjustment difficulties that are resulting from the medical symptoms and will explore whether there is a psychological component to the symptoms. He is prepared to discuss the issue further with the director and other health care providers as needed or to seek other practice opportunities if he is fired.

ALLOCATING RESOURCES

Overview

Many geropsychologists provide administrative or management functions. The settings in which such services are provided range widely and include nearly every type of setting in which older adults receive psychological services. Psychology training provides a foundation that in certain people can translate very nicely into administrative and management skills once the more specific administration and management skill set has been obtained. However, specific instruction in administrative and management skills is essentially nonexistent in psychology graduate programs, leaving clinically trained psychologists to pursue additional education on their own in business or, more commonly, to obtain the knowledge and develop the skills on the job. Attempting to apply new skills while still developing the skill set can pose ethical and professional challenges. Whereas some psychologists have excelled in the face of such challenges and become very successful in administrative and management positions, others have struggled, at times to the detriment of the institution, program, or patients. Knowledge and skills in administration and management have been described as advanced or leadership competencies in geropsychology (Knight et al., 2009).

Vignette

A geropsychologist manages the psychological services for an older adult physical medicine and rehabilitation program that is part of a larger rehabilitation program for patients of all ages. The geropsychologist reports directly to the program's overall administrator. Because of problems with reimbursement, there have been budget cuts throughout the rehabilitation program, affecting all clinical disciplines and patient populations. One day, with one staff psychologist on vacation and the other unexpectedly taking family medical leave for an unknown period of time, the geropsychologist finds herself understaffed and unable to meet the clinical needs of the patients. She discusses the issue with the administrator who advises her to assign one of the psychologists who works on the pediatric service, which has a low census at the moment, to the geropsychology service as a solution to what they hope will be a relatively short-term problem. The geropsychologist balks at the idea. However, the administrator then informs her that there are no other options and that if she does not follow his recommendation, then she needs to work overtime, with no additional pay, to provide the coverage herself. The geropsychologist takes the suggestions under advisement and then uses the opportunity to request much-needed testing materials. The administrator informs her that there are no funds for such materials and that she should try to find a creative solution to the problems, such as downloading available test materials from the Internet. After some discussion and attempts to educate the administrator about the risks of having a pediatric psychologist cover a geriatric service and the inappropriateness and illegality of downloading copyright-protected test materials from the Internet, the geropsychologist makes no headway, and the meeting ends.

Ethical Issues, Tensions, and Resources

In administrative and management positions, geropsychologists may be positioned to determine whether valuable and sometimes limited resources, including staff and materials, are allocated appropriately, consistent with the principle of justice. The ability to make such determinations effectively is linked to the geropsychologist's professional competence to handle such matters. Principle D (Justice) states, "Psychologists exercise reasonable judgment and take precautions to ensure that their potential biases, the boundaries of their competence, and the limitations of their expertise do not lead to or condone unjust practices." Many sections of the Ethics Code are applicable, including Standards 2.01, Boundaries of Competence; 2.02, Providing Services in Emergencies; 2.05, Delegation of Work to Others; 3.11, Psychological Services Delivered to or Through Organizations; and 3.12, Interruption of Psychological Services.

The geropsychologist must decide whether assigning a pediatric psychologist to the geropsychology service on a limited basis would be more helpful than harmful to the patients and whether attempting to do so would place an unreasonable demand on the pediatric psychologist. The geropsychologist's efforts to serve the older adult patients without causing them more problems pit the principles of beneficence and nonmaleficence against one another.

The geropsychologist refers to the Ethics Code; Standard 2.02, Providing Services in Emergencies, states,

> In emergencies, when psychologists provide services to individuals for whom other mental health services are not available and for which psychologists have not obtained the necessary training, psychologists may provide such services in order to ensure that services are not denied. The services are discontinued as soon as the emergency has ended or appropriate services are available.

The geropsychologist is unsure whether her situation would be considered an emergency, but failing to provide adequate coverage would certainly result in an interruption of important psychological services. Standard 3.12, Interruption of Psychological Services, addresses this topic:

> Unless otherwise covered by contract, psychologists make reasonable efforts to plan for facilitating services in the event that psychological services are interrupted by factors such as the psychologist's illness, death, unavailability, relocation or retirement or by the client's/patient's relocation or financial limitations.

Standard 2.05, Delegation of Work to Others, further states,

> Psychologists who delegate work to employees . . . take reasonable steps to . . . (2) authorize only those responsibilities that such persons can be expected to perform competently on the basis of their education, training or experience, either independently or with the level of supervision being provided; and (3) see that such persons perform these services competently.

The geropsychologist then consults an experienced colleague who has held a variety of positions in the institution in which he works and is currently in an administrative role. The colleague's experience suggests that in most situations compromises can be made that satisfy the needs of all parties for relatively short-term problems.

Preferred Course of Action

The geropsychologist decides that by rearranging her usual schedule she can probably devote some additional time to clinical and supervisory tasks, picking up a couple of the more challenging patients, decreasing or temporarily suspending services for those patients who are least in need, and asking the pediatric psychologist to take on, under her supervision, a couple of patients who need continued services but whose cases do not seem particularly complicated. Knowing her staff as she does, she is confident that the pediatric psychologist will understand the bind that the department is in and will be willing to assist. Had that not been the situation, she would have had to consider other staffing options. With a plan in place that will meet the needs of the patient and likely satisfy the administration, she decides to confront the issue of obtaining new test materials more energetically.

ADVERTISING SERVICES AND PROGRAMS

Overview

Advertising and marketing activities can help businesses educate others about their products or services, generate interest in the business, and increase the financial bottom line. Businesses owned and run by geropsychologists range from sole proprietor practices to large corporations that employ or contract with dozens or hundreds of clinicians and support staff. Like managerial and administrative knowledge and skills, "Business information in geropsychology is unfortunately often gained the hard way by trial and error" (Vacha-Haase, 2011, p. 156). It is the *error* part of the process that puts geropsychologists at risk for not achieving their otherwise high standards of ethical practice. Available resources (e.g., Hartman-Stein, 2006) can help geropsychologists minimize the errors encountered when learning the business aspects of practice and possibly experience more of a trial and accomplishment process. Good business practices and sound ethical practice are inextricably linked.

One issue that all geropsychology business owners share is a focus on the importance of generating enough revenue to cover expenses and an acceptable profit so that providing quality services to older adults remains viable. Although the personal effects of insufficient revenue may be experienced more immediately and intensely by private business owners, the same issues are experienced by geropsychologists charged with running public and nonprofit programs or facilities. Billing for clinical services has long been a primary method of generating revenue in private practices, long-term care facilities, and other settings in which psychological services are provided to older adults. Geropsychologists have been advised to "[p]ractice appropriate documentation, billing, and reimbursement procedures for geropsychological services in compliance with state and federal laws and regulations (especially regarding Medicare and Medicaid services), including assessment and documentation of medical necessity" (Knight et al., 2009, Skill Competency A7, p. 213). However, some well-meaning professionals and those with more negative intentions have not maintained adequate documentation practices.

As mentioned in Chapter 5, the Office of the Inspector General's Office of Evaluation and Inspections found that 27% of psychiatric services provided in nursing homes were medically unnecessary, with Medicare payments for such services being inappropriate (U.S. Department of Health and Human Services, Office of the Inspector General, 2001). Lack of medical necessity was commonly found (a) with patients who had such severe cognitive limitations that they were deemed, by reviewers, to be inappropriate for these services; (b) with patients who were unable to benefit from the services; (c) when there was inappropriate frequency or duration of treatment; and (d) when services did not appear to stabilize or improve patients' conditions. Psychological testing was the most problematic mental health service; 39% of the psychological tests that were administered were medically unnecessary because they were too long, administered too frequently, or not needed by the patient. While some of the inappropriate services represented intentionally fraudulent activity, some problems occurred when clinicians did not adequately document appropriate services and medical necessity and when local insurance carriers did not properly define procedures for coding psychological testing. Thus, the skill competency for billing described by Knight et al. (2009) should be taken seriously if business owners want to keep getting paid. Standard 6: Record Keeping and Fees, related guidelines (e.g., "Record keeping guidelines"; APA, 2007), insurance carrier (especially Medicare) regulations, and related laws direct psychologists regarding appropriate documentation and billing activities.

Operating a successful business involves many activities other than providing clinical services and billing for those services. Marketing one's practice or business often helps to generate referrals and can be accomplished in many ways, including written (paper or online) advertisements, presentations to various groups in the community, and networking with other professionals who are potential referral sources or business partners such as primary care practices. Additionally, basic clerical activities such as answering telephones and mail, responding to e-mail, filing and maintaining records, scheduling appointments, and providing a safe and comfortable clinical environment are tasks that the business owner performs or delegates, and all have the potential for promoting or undermining ethical practice.

Vignette

A geropsychologist retains the services of a marketing firm that promises to increase her revenue streams and thus her income by at least 25% within a year. The firm will create a website and engage in other publicity and marketing efforts to promote her practice. The geropsychologist provides some preliminary content for the website and other materials and then looks forward to viewing the final products as they are launched and otherwise rolled out. Once the website goes live and some printed materials have been generated, the geropsychologist reviews the materials and thinks that some of the claims could be a bit grandiose but that overall, everything seemed professionally done and appealing to consumers. Examples of the potentially grandiose statements include "Dr. A cures anxiety and depression in older adults in 12 sessions or less" and "Dr. A will help you stop hoarding in 8 sessions, or you pay nothing." When the geropsychologist asks the marketing director about the "paying nothing" part, the director states that the geropsychologist can just refund the copay and keep what the insurance has paid because the patient does not actually pay that part. The geropsychologist thinks that the idea is clever and innovative.

Ethical Issues, Tensions, and Resources

In the drive to promote business, geropsychologists must be mindful not to succumb to the temptation to overstate the potential benefits of their services. They may have justified enthusiasm for the contributions they can make to welfare and care of their older adult patients, but they should exercise caution: Establishing unrealistic expectations in patients or their families has the potential to result in considerable disappointment and frustration when the expectations are not met and valuable time and resources have been expended. Geropsychologists should emphasize truthfulness, accuracy, and integrity in their marketing and publicity efforts (Principle C: Integrity; Standard 5: Advertising and Other Public Statements) and their billing practices and descriptions of fees (Standard 6: Record Keeping and Fees). Geropsychologists who advertise, or pay others to market, their practices or programs, "do not make false, deceptive, or fraudulent statements" concerning their services or "the scientific or clinical basis for or results or degree of success of, their services" (Standard 5.01b, Avoidance of False or Deceptive Statements). Geropsychologists who delegate the publicity or marketing of their professional activities to others are still ultimately responsible for the content of those materials (Standard 5.02, Statements by Others). In this case, guaranteeing a successful outcome or else the psychologist returns payment sets up an unrealistic expectation and is poor practice, while refunding the co-pay and keeping what the insurance company pays is illegal. Both activities conflict with a variety of ethical principles including fidelity and responsibility (Principle B) and integrity (Principle C).

In the desire both to help older adults and to generate income, geropsychologists may struggle with how to develop publicity and marketing ideas that convey benefits of treatment that can be reasonably expected while being appealing enough to bring new clients into the office. Offering financial incentives such as discounts or refunds may seem like a good way to promote business, but there are risks of engaging in fraudulent billing practices, particularly when insurance payments are involved. In this case specifically, the ethical requirements and guidelines are generally consistent with one another that the marketing behavior is inappropriate. In general practice there is lingering tension and controversy within professional psychology regarding ethical ways to increase business.

Preferred Course of Action

The geropsychologist will benefit from being more involved with the marketing efforts, especially the "copy" that is on her website and goes out with printed materials. Having the materials reviewed by one or more trusted colleagues who are willing to provide critical feedback could reduce the potential for grandiose statements or inappropriate offers and could potentially generate new, helpful ideas for the materials.

CLARIFYING FEES AND BILLING ARRANGEMENTS

Overview

Older adults present with a variety of payment sources, including Medicare, Medicaid, private insurance carriers, no-fault insurance, attorneys, and private pay by themselves or family members. In addition, some veterans are currently able to receive services in the community that are paid for by Veterans Affairs. Each payment source involves regulations or procedures that geropsychologists must understand and follow if they accept that type of payment and hope to be paid for their services. Even for patients or their families who pay out of pocket, decisions must be made about issues such as whether to require full payment at the time of the service, accept a payment plan, require payment in advance, and become involved in helping the patient pursue reimbursement from an insurance carrier and how to provide receipts and have patients sign a form waiving their right to use Medicare. Fees and billing options, including waiving fees and offering pro bono services, have ethical, professional, and legal implications. Primary legal and ethical requirements involve understanding and following regulations and ensuring that patients or their surrogates understand and agree to the billing arrangements before services are provided or as soon thereafter as possible.

Vignette

A geropsychologist receives a call from a woman seeking a cognitive evaluation for her 85-year-old mother, whose capacity to manage finances is in question. When the caller asks about fees for the evaluation, she is informed that the initial appointment is $250, which she finds acceptable. At the conclusion of the initial appointment, on the basis of the information obtained about the patient's status and needs, the geropsychologist informs the patient and her daughter that the fee for a comprehensive decisional capacity evaluation will be $3,000, which shocks the patient and her daughter. When the geropsychologist then informs them that she does not accept Medicare or Medicaid, which is the patient's coverage, the patient and her daughter are frustrated and angry because they cannot afford to pay for the evaluation themselves. They believe they are being cheated out of the initial $250 because they would not have come for the initial appointment if they had known about the total price for the evaluation, and they refuse to pay for the initial appointment. However, they state that they will pay for the initial appointment if the geropsychologist sends the initial consultation report to another psychologist with whom they will consult. The geropsychologist refuses to release any records until paid. During the interview, the geropsychologist learned that the patient's daughter cleans homes for a living. The geropsychologist states that she will release the initial consultation report if the patient's daughter cleans her home on two occasions; otherwise, she will use a collection agency to pursue payment.

Ethical Issues, Tensions, and Resources

Standard 6.04, Fees and Financial Arrangements, section (a) states, "As early as is feasible in a professional or scientific relationship, psychologists and recipients of psychological services reach an agreement specifying compensation and billing arrangements." Although this occurred for the initial consultation appointment, the geropsychologist did not provide costs, or even a range of possible prices, for a full cognitive capacity evaluation. She also did not inform the patient's daughter in advance that she required private payment only. Such information was essential for the patient and her daughter to be able to make an informed decision about pursuing services with this practitioner. Withholding records until payment is made, because this is not an emergency situation, is acceptable according to Standard 6.03, Withholding Records for Nonpayment. Bartering with this patient and her daughter also appears to be a possible recourse according to Standard 6.05, Barter With Clients/Patients: "Barter is the acceptance of goods, services, or other nonmonetary remuneration from clients/patients in return for psychological services. Psychologists may barter only if (1) it is not clinically contraindicated, and (2) the resulting arrangement is not exploitative."

Regarding using the collection agency to obtain payment, Standard 6.04(e) states:

> If the recipient of services does not pay for services as agreed, and if psychologists intend to use collection agencies or legal measures to collect the fees, psychologists first inform the person that such measures will be taken and provide that person an opportunity to make prompt payment.

Requiring the patient's daughter to work off the services rendered to avoid use of a collection agency, rather than offering that as one possible option among a few payment options, appears exploitative, which is also inconsistent with Principle B (Fidelity and Responsibility) and Principle C (Integrity). Knight et al. (2009) stated that geropsychologists "practice appropriate documentation, billing, and reimbursement procedures for geropsychological services in compliance with state and federal laws and regulations (especially regarding Medicare and Medicaid services), including assessment and documentation of medical necessity" (p. 213).

Preferred Course of Action

The geropsychologist should have described not only her fee for the initial consultation but also the specific fee, if known, or the anticipated fee range for the complete capacity evaluation when fees were first discussed with the patient's daughter during the initial phone contact. The geropsychologist should also have informed the patient's daughter that private pay was required. Any other possible billing arrangements, such as a sliding fee scale, bartering, or extended payment plan, could also have been discussed at that time. If no acceptable fee arrangement could be reached, the geropsychologist should have considered whether she knew of any colleagues who accept the patient's insurance coverage and made appropriate referrals accordingly.

CONCLUSION

Geropsychologists commonly have professional responsibilities that extend beyond direct patient care. Such responsibilities tend to be neglected topics in graduate training and include consultation with a variety of individuals and organizations, administrative activities, and the business aspects of practice. General ethical principles and specific ethical standards inform geropsychologists about how to negotiate these responsibilities and if followed may serve all parties well, help avoid legal troubles, and promote public trust in the profession. Attention to the underlying ethical issues, while always important, tends to be of particular concern for geropsychologists assuming new, nonclinical responsibilities or making the transition from direct clinical services to administrative duties. At these times, before competence in the new role or setting is firmly established, the risk of ethical missteps is highest. Consultation with colleagues who are experienced in the new professional activity can help identify relevant ethical issues and potential challenges so that ethical problems can be avoided and high level of satisfaction with the new role can be achieved.

7

EDUCATION, TRAINING, AND RESEARCH IN GEROPSYCHOLOGY

The principle goal of education is to create [individuals] who are capable of doing new things, not simply of repeating what other generations have done.

—Jean Piaget

Publication is a marathon, not a sprint.

—Jo Linsdell

The ethical issues involved in teaching, supervision, research, and mentoring in geropsychology are multifaceted. This chapter focuses on ethical issues in the context of the design and description of training programs, accuracy in teaching, student disclosure of personal information, assessing student and supervisee performance, and academic mentoring in geropsychological research. Many geropsychologists are employed in institutions of higher education as well as in Veterans Affairs (VA) or medical practice settings in which research and program evaluation is an expected part of their job. Therefore, an in-depth understanding of research ethics is required in a wide variety of employment settings. Certain topics, such as mandatory individual or group therapy, or sexual relationships with students and supervisees, are not covered in this chapter because no unique considerations apply to the work of geropsychologists.

http://dx.doi.org/10.1037/0000010-008
Ethical Practice in Geropsychology, by S. S. Bush, R. S. Allen, and V. A. Molinari

EDUCATION AND TRAINING PROGRAMS

Overview

Geropsychologists strive to create training programs that provide the appropriate knowledge and experiences to meet the requirements for licensure and other training goals of the program (Standard 7.01, Design of Education and Training Programs). Moreover, geropsychology program directors and supervisors ensure that current and accurate descriptions of their training programs are readily available to all interested parties (Standard 7.02, Descriptions of Education and Training Programs). For example, Allen, Crowther, and Molinari (2013) described the process of academic mentoring of students pursuing a doctoral degree with focused scientist–practitioner training in geropsychology, with the Pikes Peak training model being used to define, assess, and refine competency goals and attainment (Knight, Karel, Hinrichsen, Qualls, & Duffy, 2009).

Allen, Crowther, and Molinari (2013) highlighted as an exemplar the longstanding scientist–practitioner clinical geropsychology training program at The University of Alabama. Required coursework includes lifespan development, cognition and learning, clinical aging intervention, clinical aging assessment, and advanced practicum experiences in a variety of settings. The geropsychology practicum involves individual and sometimes couples or family therapy, participation in an interdisciplinary geriatrics clinic, and opportunities for assessment experience in collaboration with the Elder Law Clinic. The Mary Starke Harper Geriatric Psychiatry Center offers a 20-hours-per-week paid placement. Additional voluntary placement opportunities, which include local community-based and VA hospice programs (both inpatient and outpatient), are also available to students in the geropsychology program. A grant from the Graduate Geropsychology Education program (2003–2006) sponsored by the federal Health Resources and Services Administration supplemented university funding and enabled program enhancements that were then evaluated through the lens of the Pikes Peak training model (Wharton, Shah, Scogin, & Allen, 2013).

Geropsychologists in academia and clinical training settings are committed to being effective educators. They are committed not just to meeting basic ethical requirements, such as having syllabi reflecting accurate course content and rendering course material current (Standard 7.03, Accuracy in Teaching); they strive to advance their skills as educators (Standard 2.03, Maintaining Competence) and to convey their abilities as educators to their students and trainees. Many institutions of higher learning provide some form of teaching of graduate students about teaching. Unfortunately, a recent survey of geropsychology graduate students and postdoctoral fellows revealed that teaching training lags behind research training, and such a state of affairs is particularly concerning because of the geropsychology workforce shortage (Carpenter, Sakai, Karel, Molinari, & Moye, 2016).

Tenure-track faculty members frequently are encouraged to seek mentorship in high-quality teaching from senior colleagues who have been recognized for their teaching excellence. However, it is rare for university settings to provide formal mentorship opportunities for junior faculty. Junior geropsychology faculty members at universities that offer a Teaching of Psychology class (Rickard, Prentice-Dunn, Rogers, Scogin, & Lyman, 1991) but have never taken such a course may advance their competence in teaching by sitting in on the class along with the graduate students who are enrolled in the course. Thorough didactic and experiential knowledge of "teaching of teaching" facilitates geropsychologists in designing and implementing high-quality education and training programs (Standard 7.01, Design of Education and Training Programs).

A Teaching of Psychology class has been offered at The University of Alabama since 1974, designed to replace a written comprehensive examination yet also to fulfill the need for graduate students to integrate their knowledge of psychology. Junior faculty occasionally "sit in" on the class or consult with the professor, an exemplary teacher, to enhance their own professional teaching skills (Standard 2.03, Maintaining Competence). The class is constructed such that, in addition to having primary responsibility for a section of Introductory Psychology with limited enrollment, students attend a 2-hour weekly seminar on teaching that incorporates active learning techniques such as videotaping, consultation, and peer review. McElroy and Prentice-Dunn (2005) examined the feedback of 36 graduate students enrolled in similar Teaching of Psychology courses in two universities and found that graduate students reported that reviewing videotapes of their teaching with the course instructor and consultation with the instructor about undergraduate student ratings of teaching were integral to the value of the course.

Vignette

A geropsychology graduate student in a Teaching of Psychology class, taught by an exemplary teacher and full professor, planned a lecture in his introductory course regarding healthy aging and sexuality. Clearly stated in the course syllabus was one lecture devoted to film clips from the documentary *Still Doing It: The Intimate Lives of Women Over 60* (Fishel, 2004) followed by planned class discussion; a thorough description of the video and the URL address were provided on the syllabus. This course content had been thoroughly considered and vetted by the geropsychology graduate student, the professor, and the other graduate psychology students enrolled in the Teaching of Psychology course. The geropsychology graduate student took care to mention in class and through the course website that this course content would be presented soon and that any undergraduate students who did not wish to attend this lecture or be exposed to this content could instead read a brief scientific article about healthy aging and write a two-page report. Despite this careful preparation, the geropsychology graduate student, course instructor, and chairperson of the psychology department received a complaint from an undergraduate student and his mother that such course content represented unethical and pornographic material that had no business in the college classroom. After careful review, the department chair met with the undergraduate student and his mother to attempt to allay concerns but also reinforce the idea that the geropsychology graduate student and course instructor had behaved in accordance with usual and customary educational practices and professional ethics (Standard 7.03, Accuracy in Teaching).

Ethical Decision-Making Process

As illustrated in Exhibits 3.1 and 3.2, a sequence of ethical decision-making questions and steps provides a structured approach to addressing ethical challenges. Asking oneself the questions and following the steps for each case is likely to help achieve good outcomes.

Ethical Issues, Tensions, and Resources

Perceptions and expectations differ regarding which behaviors and disclosures by a graduate student with primary responsibility for an introductory course exemplify accuracy and appropriateness in teaching (Standard 7.03, Accuracy in Teaching) and which can be harmful to undergraduate students in the classroom and should be avoided (Standard 3.04, Avoiding Harm). In this case, the geropsychology graduate student, course instructor, and department chair demonstrated sensitivity to differing values. They believed that by providing information in the syllabus, classroom, and course website regarding the content of the documentary on healthy sexual expression in women over age 60 and by providing an alternative educational opportunity requiring similar time and effort, they had made sufficient effort to avoid harm to the undergraduate student.

Preferred Course of Action

In this scenario, the geropsychology graduate student followed the preferred course of action by clearly discussing inclusion of the healthy aging and sexuality course content with the professor and fellow students prior to listing the documentary on his course syllabus. Moreover, an accurate description of video content to be shown in class was provided in the syllabus, during classroom lecture, and an alternative assignment also was provided on the course website. After the negative reaction by the undergraduate student and his mother, the preferred course of action for the geropsychology graduate student was to refer the complaint to the course professor and department chair and then to refrain from actively engaging the undergraduate student or his parent in further discussion of the issue so that the complaint could "work its way through proper channels." Academic freedom, an essential tenet of higher education, facilitates the mission of the academic institution by encouraging freedom of inquiry by faculty members. Within ethical boundaries, scholars and educators, including mentored students, should have freedom to teach or communicate controversial ideas or facts without being targeted for retaliation or job loss, even when those ideas or facts may be unpopular or subject to discrimination or bias. Adverse effects, including numerous student complaints or evidence of harassment or unfair discrimination, would be needed to justify superseding academic freedom and discontinuing use of the video.

STUDENT AND TRAINEE PERFORMANCE

Overview

Teaching and supervision of students in geropsychology requires building a strong mentoring relationship and ongoing clear communication with the student and others in the training program. All graduate programs have guidelines regarding academic and nonacademic failure. Standard 7.04, Student Disclosure of Personal Information, states that programs do not require student disclosure of personal information except when the program clearly identifies this as a requirement or personal problems could reasonably be judged to be interfering with the student's academic or professional performance. The latter exception could lead to nonacademic failure and may result in a wide variety of ways in which performance standards are not met, including problems with (a) completing psychotherapy notes or assessment reports on time, (b) attendance at meetings with clinical supervisors, (c) attendance at clinical placement sites, (d) careful and confidential handling of assessment or therapy material regarding a client, and (e) poor assessment and treatment performance resulting from barriers in therapeutic rapport or ability to effectively implement assessment and or treatment protocols. Such circumstances require clear informal and formal communication with the student and, eventually, documentation in the student's record. Corrective remediation plans are typical and consist of specific behavioral performance guidelines within a specified timeline. If corrective remediation plans are sufficiently implemented and the student responds appropriately, the student may avoid formal probation, which must be documented in the student's record and reported to any potential internship sites. Judgment of successfully meeting the conditions of a corrective remediation plan requires assessing student or supervisee performance until it is deemed satisfactory (Standard 7.06, Assessing Student and Supervisee Performance).

With regard to assessing geropsychology students' teaching performance, Prentice-Dunn (2006) provided the following guidelines: (a) give the student explicit permission to be imperfect (expect improvement but not perfection as teaching skills develop across time and experience), (b) shape students' expectations of the teaching experience through readings, (c) encourage students' early use of several teaching techniques, and (d) use active learning exercises in Teaching of Psychology courses. Prentice-Dunn also recommended a collaborative rather than expert approach to teaching graduate students how to teach, including (a) use of multiple sources of feedback, (b) structure of consultation sessions to focus student attention on important points, and (c) help in recognizing the rhythms of the semester. Prentice-Dunn, Payne, and Ledbetter (2006) recommended specific behaviors for structured consultation sessions between the graduate student and experienced instructor: (a) ask the graduate student to take the lead in discussion of his or her teaching, (b) focus on positive behaviors first, (c) frame problems in terms of areas for improvement, and (d) help the student set short-term teaching goals. These specific guidelines can be used to ethically assess graduate students' performance in learning how to teach (Standard 7.06, Assessing Student and Supervisee Performance).

With regard to assessing students' clinical performance, the Pikes Peak self-assessment tool is useful for students, interns, and individuals at any stage in their career to evaluate their competencies based on the aspirational guidelines developed from the Pikes Peak model (Karel, Knight, Duffy, Hinrichsen, & Zeiss, 2010). The tables and example milestones provided by Molinari (2012) further assist in determining whether the knowledge- and skills-based competencies delineated in the Pikes Peak training model are being met for assessment, intervention, consultation, research, supervision training, and management and administration. To perform with the highest ethical standards, geropsychologists must also develop competencies related to work in interdisciplinary teams and knowledge of relevant public policies that affect older individuals (Molinari, 2012; O'Shea Carney, Gum, & Zeiss, 2015).

Knight (2010) described processes of clinical supervision for assessment and psychotherapy with older adults, noting that the scope of supervision may be broader because of the heterogeneity of issues experienced by older adults and the interdisciplinary nature of these issues. Knight recommended that geropsychologists may meet the highest ethical standards in the evaluation of student performance by (a) helping trainees remain aware of the hypothetical nature of initial diagnoses and treatment plans, (b) assisting trainees in evaluating the applicability of assessment instruments to special populations, (c) maintaining awareness of both positive and negative age stereotypes in supervision, and (d) recognizing that substance abuse may be an issue among older adults. Over the course of supervision with trainees, geropsychologists should incorporate information regarding issues such as cohort competency (knowledge of the historical events older adults have encountered), cultural competency, knowledge of "who is the client," handling comments regarding client–student age differential, and tactics about how to effectively and respectfully interrupt or confront older adult clients. These activities foster effective supervision. Because preparation for supervision is varied in graduate and postdoctoral geropsychology programs and there is a general need for more training in supervision (Karel, Sakai, Molinari, Moye, & Carpenter, 2016), geropsychologists who are becoming, or plan to become, supervisors have a responsibility to supplement their formal supervision training, or lack thereof, with self-study and consultation with experienced colleagues.

Vignette

An African American geropsychology graduate student brings the following incident to supervision. The student has been conducting home-based psychoeducational and behavioral activation therapy with an 82-year-old non-Hispanic White widowed woman receiving palliative care for congestive heart failure at her daughter's home. The patient has suffered a series of strokes leaving her with moderate cognitive impairment and physical limitations. The patient also is morbidly obese and confined to her bed. Her daughter is a substitute middle school teacher and occasionally leaves the patient at home alone when she substitute teaches. The daughter always leaves the house telephone within her mother's reach and alerts a neighbor to the possibility that her mother will call during the school day if the need arises. The geropsychology graduate student has been educating the patient's daughter about caregiving issues, including the risks that leaving her mother home alone presents and the potential need for respite care. The student also has been working with the mother (the patient) to reduce symptoms of depression.

The geropsychology student reports to the supervisory group that, on one occasion, the home health aide arrived at the home to find the patient had been incontinent and was covered in her own feces. The patient reported that she had called out for her daughter, but her daughter did not appear to be home. The telephone sat beside the patient on a bedstand. Despite her daughter's lack of availability at times, the patient does not want to live anywhere else. The home health aide provided continence care and bathed the patient, who reiterated her commitment and desire to continue living with her daughter. The home health aide then reported the incident to her supervisor, and the issue was discussed in the interdisciplinary team meeting, which was attended by the geropsychology student. The geropsychology student wonders whether there is a responsibility to do more to help this patient, and she discusses this issue with her supervisor at their next scheduled supervisory appointment.

Ethical Issues, Tensions, and Resources

Consistent with Principle A (Beneficence and Nonmaleficence), the geropsychology student has an obligation to promote the safety and well-being of the patient, such as by intervening with the patient's daughter to explain her mother's need for greater support in meeting basic care needs as a result of her cognitive impairment and immobility. If the patient's daughter continues to be neglectful in her care of the patient, additional steps to protect the patient, such as arranging for more comprehensive coverage by home health aides or reporting the situation to Adult Protective Services, may be necessary. The geropsychology student's timely report of the incident to her supervision group reflects professional responsibility. Consideration of the patient's stated preference to remain in her daughter's care must be respected (Principle E: Respect for People's Rights and Dignity; American Psychological Association [APA], 2010), although her capacity to make such a decision may need to be clarified.

The design of educational and training programs such as the one in which the graduate student is enrolled must include specific procedures for trainees who encounter clinical issues of potential abuse or neglect among their older adult clients to report these situations to their licensed supervisor (Standard 7.01, Design of Education and Training Programs). How a student manages such circumstances in routine clinical work has direct relevance for assessing the student's performance (Standard 7.06, Assessing Student and Supervisee Performance).

Tension exists between respect for the patient's wishes and the maintenance of her autonomy (reflected in Principle E: Respect for People's Rights and Dignity) and beneficence on the part of the interdisciplinary treatment team that wants to ensure her safety, and these issues should be an area of focus with the geropsychology student during supervision. Perhaps the most prominent issue to discuss in supervision is the need to report the incident as potentially representing neglect on the part of the patient's daughter. The supervisor must discuss with the geropsychology student the potential implications of reporting the incident to Adult Protective Services, including the possible repercussions for the person who does the reporting. Because the geropsychology student has an established relationship providing psychoeducation on dementia care to the patient's daughter and behavioral activation to the patient for symptoms of depression, it may be best for a member of the home health care team other than the geropsychology student to report the incident.

Preferred Course of Action

In this case, the student acted in an ethically appropriate manner by reporting the incident to the supervisor, but because this case also illustrates neglect, the student should have reported the incident to her supervisor immediately rather than waiting for scheduled supervision. The geropsychology student needed to listen carefully during the interdisciplinary team meeting, take the issue to her geropsychology supervisor in a timely manner, and learn about ethical and legal requirements, including mandatory reporting. It would be inappropriate to ignore the health risk to the patient caused by the fecal incontinence when the client's daughter works outside the home without providing in-house supervision for her mother's needs. When determining who, if anyone, would report the situation to Adult Protective Services, the harm that could be done to the therapeutic relationship with the student if the student or the supervisor were to report the incident, coupled with the advantage of the student's continued involvement with the patient and her daughter, suggests that cooperating with members of the home health care team in reporting the incident may be the best course of action (Standard 3.09, Cooperation With Other Professionals).

ACADEMIC MENTORING AND GRANTSMANSHIP

Overview

In the scientist–practitioner training model, the goal is for the areas in which students provide clinical service to inform their research and vice versa (Gelso, 2006). This link between research and clinical activities facilitates but does not guarantee both evidence-based practice and practice-based evidence translatable to the real world. Specific research goals for trainees may include (a) developing a research program based on the trainee's interest and learning objectives; (b) learning research and professional skills, including how to obtain approval from institutional review boards (IRBs) and collect primary data; (c) publishing empirical journal articles, book chapters, and other material (e.g., encyclopedia entries, systematic literature reviews); (d) developing a competitive curriculum vitae and expertise to acquire a desired academic job after completion of training; and (e) developing and submitting collaborative grant or contract proposals if appropriate to the trainee's interests (Phillips, Fisher, Allen, & Burgio, 2004). Each of these goals is facilitated by effective mentorship.

The classic definition of a *mentor* is someone of advanced rank and experience who guides, teaches, and develops a novice. Zerzan, Hess, Schur, Phillips, and Rigotti (2009) defined *mentoring* as "a symbiotic relationship aimed at advancing careers and career satisfaction for both the mentor and the mentee. Ideally, it is a dynamic, collaborative, reciprocal relationship focused on a mentee's personal and professional development" (p. 140). Mentoring occurs within career-focused and personal or psychosocial domains (Clark, Harden, & Johnson, 2000; Straus, Johnson, Marquez, & Feldman, 2013; Zerzan et al., 2009). Career functions include sponsoring, networking, coaching, protecting, and providing challenging collaborative work assignments. Psychosocial functions operate at the interpersonal level and include role modeling, acceptance and affirmation, career counseling, and friendship. Within the field of geropsychology, mentoring involves issues particular to working with older adults and their families and occurs in practice, research, and teaching domains. It involves building a relationship between the faculty member(s) and the student or trainee that is focused on fostering and developing the trainee's interests, enhancing and expanding skills, and promoting gradual independence through incremental steps (Phillips et al., 2004). A trainee may have multiple mentors or different primary mentors in different academic or professional domains.

Trainees start their programs at diverse places in their professional trajectory and with varying levels of experience. For example, some individuals begin graduate school immediately after graduating with a bachelor's degree, others begin after one or several years of work experience, and others begin their doctoral education with a master's degree or other professional degree and ample prior work experience (e.g., social work or nursing). Typically, trainees move immediately from a graduate program to an internship and then, frequently, into postdoctoral training (Allen, Crowther, & Molinari, 2013). Zerzan and colleagues (2009) advised mentees to take an active role in the mentoring relationship throughout their professional trajectory. They recommended seeking mentors early and in multiple places both inside and outside of one's own institution. They further recommended seeking mentors who are both junior- and senior-level colleagues in order to receive advice that is proximal and distal to one's own goals and current state of development. Unfortunately, the number of bona fide geropsychologists remains small, and mentors may be difficult to find in specific graduate school and internship settings. Geropsychology organizations such as Psychologists in Long Term Care and the American Board of Geropsychology have therefore begun to implement their own mentoring programs. Moreover, organizations such as APA's Society of Clinical Geropsychology and the Council of Professional Geropsychology Training Programs provide opportunities for graduate students and trainees to become involved with organizational activities and receive informal and formal mentorship from geropsychologists.

Straus and colleagues (2013) conducted a qualitative study of the characteristics of successful and unsuccessful mentoring relationships. Using grounded theory to analyze interviews with 54 faculty members at two academic health centers (one in the United States and one in Canada), the authors identified characteristics of successful mentoring relationships, shown in Exhibit 7.1.

Throughout the course of training for a potential academic career in a university or medical school, geropsychologists may well face the daunting task of writing and submitting grant applications to external funding sources or various foundations and other granting agencies. Geropsychologists may mentor students or other trainees in seeking external funding through dissertation grants (e.g., Individual Predoctoral Fellows awards, Health Services Research Dissertation Awards) or career development awards. One primary goal in academic medical centers and universities frequently is to teach grantsmanship (Phillips et al., 2004).

Notably, students cannot directly receive funds from most granting agencies through "R mechanisms" because these grants require the principal investigator to have a terminal degree. However, occasionally students or other trainees or even junior faculty may function as project managers and co-principal investigators on projects led by senior faculty. These junior colleagues may even contribute heavily to the grant writing process (Phillips et al., 2004). Particularly when a junior colleague's career goal is to obtain tenure in an academic position, gaining experience through applying for grant funding in a mentored way can be extremely valuable (a) to be optimally prepared for an academic research career and competitive in the academic market, (b) to contribute to the larger body of research and clinical knowledge, (c) to collaborate

EXHIBIT 7.1
Characteristics of Successful and Unsuccessful Mentoring Relationships

Successful	Unsuccessful
Reciprocity between mentors and mentees	Poor communication
Mutual respect	Lack of commitment
Clear expectations	Personality differences between the mentor and mentee
Personal connection	Perceived (or real) competition
Shared values	Conflicts of interest including different agendas for the mentor and mentee
	Lack of experience of the mentor

Note. Data from Straus, Johnson, Marquez, and Feldman (2013).

and network with other top researchers in a specific area of geropsychology, and (d) to secure independent funding for a specific period of further training (Phillips et al., 2004).

There are ethical implications for mentoring of grant applications and other scholarly activities. The *Ethical Principles of Psychologists and Code of Conduct* (APA, 2010; hereinafter referred to as the Ethics Code) clearly describes standards regarding human relations (Standard 3: Human Relations) that are pertinent to the research and publication process (Standard 8: Research and Publication) and reflective of successful mentoring relationships. The following case illustration, however, describes how such relationships may go awry.

Vignette

After receiving her master's degree, a doctoral student began studies in geropsychology under the mentorship of a new tenure-track assistant professor. The student and mentor were close in age and shared interests in healthy aging and sport psychology. Both women were also members of the local track club in the small town. At first, they developed a close mentoring relationship due to their shared professional and personal interests. As they spent time together professionally and personally, however, difficulties arose in their relationship because of conflicts of interest. The student's stated goal was to complete her doctoral training within 3 years; thus, her agenda for completing coursework, accruing enough varied clinical hours for internship, and completing her doctoral dissertation put her on a "fast track" in graduate school. Her mentor, meanwhile, greatly valued the student's skill set, contribution to her own healthy aging laboratory, and friendship. The mentor kept emphasizing to the student that the average graduate student required 4 to 5 years to complete the doctoral training before leaving for internship. Moreover, the mentor really wanted the student to stay in the program for 4 years because the priority score and percentile ranking of the grant they submitted in the student's first year of graduate study was likely to be funded. The student considered this grant her dissertation, whereas her mentor saw it as one step in a shared collaborative research program. The student began to feel as if the mentor did not have her best interests in mind and to believe that her mentor was taking advantage of her.

Ethical, Issues, Tensions, and Resources

Although the mentoring relationship likely started with a personal connection related to shared interests, reciprocity, and mutual respect, the communication about professional aspirations was not optimal, given that expectations between the mentor and mentee were not clear (see Exhibit 7.1). The ethical tensions in this scenario vary based on the perspective of the individual involved. Although the mentor likely did not perceive her interactions with the student as exploitive (Standard 3.08: Exploitative Relationships), it appears that the student grew to perceive them as such. This is particularly true of the apparent disagreement regarding the purpose and "ownership" of the submitted research grant. Only faculty members, not student trainees, can be listed as principal investigators of this type of grant mechanism, adding to the potential complexity of the ethical issues depending on the level of involvement the student had in writing the grant application.

Straus and colleagues (2013) emphasized the importance of setting clear expectations in the formation of successful mentoring relationships. Standard 3.05, Multiple Relationships, advises psychologists to resolve a potentially harmful relationship with due regard to the best interests of the affected person when unforeseen factors causing "multiple relationships" arise. Standard 3.06, Conflict of Interest, advises psychologists to refrain from taking on professional roles when personal, professional, scientific, or financial issues arise that may impair their objectivity. It seems that the student and her mentor had different perceptions of whether their relationship became exploitive.

Preferred Course of Action

The likely preferred course of action would be for the director of clinical/counseling training to become involved and mediate a mutually agreeable solution. It may be that the student will need to find another primary mentor, though she will likely want to remain involved if the research grant should be funded, to progress along her chosen career path. Moreover, the mentor would likely benefit from mentoring by senior colleagues (e.g., associate or full professors) about the benefits and challenges of developing close personal friendships with trainees.

IRBS AND PROTECTION OF VULNERABLE OLDER ADULTS

Overview

The U.S. Department of Health and Human Services (HHS) requires that every institution engaged in human subjects research not otherwise exempt and supported by HHS must have an approved assurance of compliance with the HHS regulations for the protection of human subjects. As a result of a series of highly publicized abuses in research ethics (e.g., Willowbrook Study 1963–1966, Rivera, 1972; Tuskegee Syphilis Study 1932–1972, Centers for Disease Control and Prevention, 2016), the HHS revised and expanded its regulations in the late 1970s and early 1980s, requiring basic protections for human subjects involved in both biomedical and behavioral research conducted or supported by HHS. Based on the Belmont Report and other work of the National Commission, three fundamental ethical principles for all human subjects research have been identified: respect for persons, beneficence, and justice. In 1991, the Federal Policy for the Protection of Human Subjects, informally known as the Common Rule, was issued by 15 federal departments and agencies (U.S. Department of Health & Human Services, 2016a). This resulted in the growth and further regulation of IRBs. Certain members of IRBs may represent specific vulnerable populations (e.g., pregnant women, prisoners, children). A professional with expertise in forensic settings may become an IRB member to represent the interests of prisoners. Older adults are not considered vulnerable based solely on their age but may be deemed so based on limitations commonly associated with advanced age, such as cognitive deficits and significantly compromised health.

Institutions must comply with regulations of the Office for Human Research Protections; the office facilitates protection of the rights, welfare, and well-being of human subjects by providing clarification and guidance, developing educational programs and materials, maintaining regulatory oversight, and offering advice on ethical and regulatory issues in biomedical and social-behavioral research. Many institutions have separate IRBs for medical and social-behavioral research, each composed of scientific and nonscientific members.

Research regarding the functioning of IRBs has produced interesting findings. Dziak and colleagues (2005) examined records of IRB applications and correspondence for a multisite (15 primary care clinics) study of health care quality involving telephone interviews with 3,000 participants. They found variations in the type of IRB required and the number of days from submission to approval (range = 5–172 days). In contrast, the VA, which employs many geropsychologists, has one central office or IRB that serves all VA settings. Perhaps partially because of research showing variability in the functioning of IRBs (Dziak et al., 2005), there is growing institutional interest nationally in seeking and obtaining accreditation by The Association for the Accreditation of Human Research Protection Programs; such accreditation provides one means of evaluating whether medical facilities and institutions of higher learning meet rigorous standards for ethics, quality, and protections for human subjects research.

Depending on the scope and nature of the research being conducted, geropsychologists, faculty, and student investigators may apply for exempt, expedited, or full board reviews. Exempt reviews must be no more than minimal risk, defined by the federal regulations as the probability and magnitude of physical or psychological harm that is normally encountered in the daily lives or in the routine medical, dental, or psychological examination of healthy persons. Depending on the institution, these reviews may be conducted by Office of Research Compliance staff or an experienced member of the IRB. Examples of geropsychological research that may qualify for exempt status include analysis of previously collected and de-identified data (e.g., large national probability studies such as the Health and Retirement Study), education research, public observations that do not involve children, or studies of public officials or service programs.

Expedited reviews are conducted by at least one experienced member of the IRB, must pose no more than minimal risk, and fall into at least one of the expedited categories defined by federal regulations. For most geropsychologists, research activities would likely fall into expedited categories 5 (research involving materials or documents that have been collected or will be collected solely for nonresearch purposes, such as treatment records), 6 (data from voice, video, digital, or image recordings made for research purposes), and 7 (research on individual or group characteristics or behavior or research employing survey, interview, oral history, focus group, program evaluation, human factors evaluation, or quality assurance methodologies; U.S. Department of Health and Human Services, 2016b). However, geropsychologists interested in research with vulnerable older adults, such as those with diminished capacity or receiving palliative or hospice care, should expect that their research will require full board approval.

Full board reviews are required when research is greater than minimal risk or does not qualify for expedited review (e.g., vulnerable populations are involved). Specific procedures in determining the need for full board review vary by site (Dziak et al., 2005). Typically, a primary reviewer is assigned for each protocol undergoing full board review, and that individual leads discussion of the protocol at a convened meeting of the IRB that includes both scientific and nonscientific members as well as any members representing vulnerable populations.

Faculty and students applying for any type of IRB approval for a research study at any institution must pay strict attention to Standards 6.01, 6.02, and 8.01 through 8.08 of the Ethics Code. For example, undergraduates completing an honor's thesis or first-year graduate students completing a First-Year Project likely develop research questions and methodologies with heavy input from the faculty mentor. In research mentorship, the training goal is for the faculty mentor (a) to embrace the student's prior research interests; (b) to foster the development of an independent line of research for the student; and (c) to provide the opportunity for students to develop skills necessary for conducting an independent research program, publication, and, perhaps, grantsmanship. Frequently, incoming students join existing projects within a lab. This allows students to learn a specific setting's IRB system and to develop community collaborations while becoming an active, contributing member of their new lab.

Special considerations are involved in training students to conduct research with vulnerable populations (e.g., cognitively impaired older adults, individuals in rural areas, prisoners) or research using deception. For example, conducting research in rural areas in which privacy may be compromised by social networks that rapidly disseminate information about individuals has special implications involving Standards 4.04, Minimizing Intrusions on Privacy; 6.01, Documentation of Professional and Scientific Work and Maintenance of Records; 6.02, Maintenance, Dissemination, and Disposal of Confidential Records of Professional and Scientific Work; and 8.02, Informed Consent to Research. In some rural areas, participation in research may conflict with local norms against research (i.e., "being a guinea pig") that developed from historical abuses or distrust of medical centers or universities. This social norm may impose greater than minimal social or psychological risk to research participants who are concerned about the protection of their privacy in small rural areas. The following case example illustrates ethical issues in research with cognitively impaired older adults who are civilly committed to an inpatient psychiatric facility.

Vignette

As part of a dissertation project, a doctoral student and her mentor are collaborating on a multisite reminiscence and creative activity randomized controlled trial aiming to increase behavioral activation among geriatric psychiatry patients who are involuntarily hospitalized in two state hospitals. To conduct this treatment outcome study, three separate IRB approvals are needed, one from each of the state hospitals and one from the university in which they work.

To be able to document their commitment to the protection of human subjects in this project, the student, her mentor, and their research team across sites read, discuss, and revisit the ethical issues addressed in an article by Testa and West (2010), which describes the history of involuntary psychiatric hospitalization in the United States. For example, on research team conference calls, participants discuss the article's coverage of all five principles of the APA (2010) Ethics Code. Testa and West also clearly described the two state laws pertaining to involuntary hospitalization: *parens patriae* and police power. *Parens patriae* refers to a doctrine of English common law in which the government is described as having the responsibility to intervene on behalf of citizens who cannot act in their own best interests. Police power requires a state to protect the interests of its citizens. The student and her mentor become experts in the issues surrounding civil commitment and decide to include a reference to the Testa and West article in each of their three IRB applications. The protocol undergoes full board review by all three IRBs.

The three IRBs involved in approving the randomized controlled trial produce different outcomes with regard to the study protocol consent procedures and methodology. Specifically, because the psychiatric inpatients are civilly committed and thus considered prisoners, the prison representative at the university voices concerns about multiple relationships, conflicts of interest, exploitative relationships, documentation of professional and scientific work and maintenance of records, and client–patient, student, and subordinate research participants. First and foremost, the prison representative is concerned that the individuals at each site who will be providing services in the treatment arm of the randomized controlled trial are students on paid practicum placements at each of the state hospitals. Therefore, these individuals are the same as those providing treatment as usual to the control group and could unduly influence their patients to participate in the research. Second, concerns about de-identification and transport of medical records information and data between the state hospitals and the university are expressed. Although the protocol is approved by the IRBs at each of the state hospitals within 30 days, responses to the university IRB result in a lag of 179 days between initial submission and eventual approval of the protocol.

Ethical Issues, Tensions, and Resources

First, the student's and mentor's motivation in conducting the randomized controlled trial is to discover whether enhanced therapeutic programming might increase the behavioral activation of geriatric inpatients and thereby result in improved mood and functioning (beneficence). The investigators diligently train themselves and their team in the ethical considerations surrounding work with individuals who are involuntarily hospitalized. However, additional issues such as potential undue influence of these vulnerable patients, considered prisoners, by the students involved in both the research protocol and provision of clinical services on paid placement at the state hospitals required additional consideration to avoid harming the patients (nonmaleficence). Specifically, psychologists "are alert to and guard against personal, financial, social, organizational, or political factors that might lead to misuse of their influence" (Principle A: Beneficence and Nonmaleficence, Ethics Code; APA, 2010). In this situation, there is concern about students acting as service providers in the setting also working to recruit participants for the clinical trial. Standard 8.04, Client/Patient, Student, and Subordinate Research Participants, states that psychologists who conduct research with clients/patients take steps to protect them from adverse consequences of declining or withdrawing from the study. The concern of the university IRB members was to balance access to a potentially beneficial treatment for psychiatric inpatients with the potential for patients to feel coerced or that their usual treatment was threatened if they did not participate in the research (Principle E: Respect for People's Rights and Dignity).

In this case, Principle D (Justice) also must be considered: "Psychologists recognize that fairness and justice entitle all persons to access to and benefit from the contributions of psychology and to equal quality in the processes, procedures and services being conducted by psychologists." Reminiscence and behavioral activation through creative activities are evidence-based effective treatments and, therefore, questions about access by all geriatric psychiatry patients to this treatment must be considered (i.e., delayed treatment control group rather than treatment as usual so that all patients may eventually receive treatment).

Materials reviewed included the Ethics Code, information provided by the Treatment Advocacy Center (2015), and the article by Testa and West (2010). The center publishes summaries of U.S. civil commitment laws by state that may be helpful for researchers in developing treatment projects in these settings. Moreover, access to better treatment standards and reports on specific diagnoses (e.g., schizophrenia) or conditions (e.g., homelessness) and approaches to dealing with stigma are available on this site.

Preferred Course of Action

In this scenario, a preferred course of action would be for student and mentor to convene an initial meeting with the chairpersons of all three IRBs (two state hospitals and the university). In a virtual or face-to-face meeting with sufficient detail to consider the ethical concerns involved, a thorough and yet expeditious plan of action might have been developed to better coordinate the three independent IRB reviews of this multisite application (Dziak et al., 2005). Such a meeting may have circumvented the nearly 6-month delay in eventual approval of this protocol by all three IRBs.

CONSENT IN RESEARCH

Overview

When IRB approval is obtained for a primary data collection project, geropsychologists must turn their attention to the ethics of actually recruiting and securing consent from participants and conducting the research. Like a variety of other populations, individuals with impaired cognition, which may result in diminished decision-making capacity, are considered a vulnerable population. Extra cautionary steps must be taken to ensure that older adult participants who may have compromised cognitive abilities have the capacity to consent to the research. Consensus recommendations for the informed consent process with individuals with diminished capacity have been provided by the Alzheimer's Association (2004) and the joint effort of the American Bar Association and the APA Assessment of Capacity in Older Adults Project Working Group (2008). To determine capacity to consent, geropsychologists assess the individual's ability (a) to understand the nature of the research and of participation (e.g., by asking participants to repeat back in their own words what the study is about); (b) to appreciate the consequences of participation (i.e., spontaneously provide both negative and positive potential consequences of participating); (c) to understand alternatives, including the option not to participate; and (d) to make a reasoned and consistent choice (i.e., provide logical reasons for wanting to participate that are consistent over time). Geropsychologists stop several times during the consent procedure to test for the individual's understanding by requesting that the person "put it into your own words." Geropsychologists reassess consent–assent at each assessment or intervention contact with older adults with diminished decision-making capacity.

The principle of justice entails consideration by geropsychologists of sampling procedures that facilitate equal access to potentially beneficial research rather than simply recruiting convenience samples. For example, if people with severe dementia were automatically excluded from research because they did not have the capacity to consent, then no studies could be conducted on this group. As in the case of any vulnerable population, the principle of justice guides geropsychologists to conduct research on the population so that their best interests will be served in the long run by getting more information about the disease process that will ultimately help them. Researchers would need to identify their legal guardians or durable powers of attorney to determine whether they would agree to the vulnerable person's research participation when using the substituted judgment or best interests criteria (Hays & Jennings, 2015). However, it should be noted that attempts to garner the potential research participant's assent to participate is also required. In this endeavor, geropsychologists may consider the principles of community-based participatory research (CBPR; Israel et al., 1998, 2010) to recruit participants from rural or other underresourced and underrepresented communities. CBPR principles also facilitate Principle E (Respect for People's Rights and Dignity) by promoting integration of community norms into research to protect individuals' privacy, confidentiality, and right to self-determination. Models that incorporate community engagement in the planning and implementation of research, particularly research into health promotion or disease prevention, have been shown to reduce the gap between dissemination of research findings in scientific and community circles. Community engagement is now recognized as having value in the translation of science (Israel et al., 1998, 2010).

With regard to education and training in research theory and activities beyond participant recruitment and consent, geropsychologists mentor students and other trainees in the ethical analysis and interpretation of research data. Beginning graduate students may receive a great deal of mentoring in conducting statistical analyses, but the student is responsible for fully understanding the analyses and developing the skills necessary to conduct analyses independently in their future research (Standard 2.01, Boundaries of Competence). Typically, a matriculating graduate student supervised by a geropsychologist attempts to create an independent line of research, from an initial First-Year Project that may entail heavy reliance on the mentor's research and projects conducted by other members of the research lab, to a relatively independent dissertation proposal. Ideally, the line of research from the First-Year Project through the master's thesis and onto the dissertation is similar so that continuity of research questions and, hopefully, findings through multiple studies begins to build (Phillips et al., 2004). Throughout this process the geropsychologist ensures that each student or trainee, approached as an individual with unique needs, interests, and strengths, thoroughly learns to apply the Ethics Code to work with human subjects and the research and scientific enterprise, either as a consumer or originator of knew knowledge, depending on the training model.

Vignette

As part of a dissertation examining cognitive capacity to execute an estate will, a doctoral student and his mentor incorporate extensive procedures recommended by the Alzheimer's Association (2004) and the handbook *Assessment of Older Adults With Diminished Capacity* (American Bar Association/APA Assessment of Capacity in Older Adults Project Working Group, 2008) to assess individuals' capacity to consent to research. They also use CBPR principles to identify a sample representative of their local medical center. Data collected routinely in the geriatrics clinic reveal that the typical patient achieves scores on a cognitive screening instrument in ranges consistent with mild neurocognitive disorders.

The student is attempting to gain the informed consent of a local resident of an assisted living facility who is also a patient in the geriatrics clinic for a research project involving capacity to complete an estate will. He notes during the consent process that the individual is able to restate the goal of the research and has a basic understanding of the research procedure and what an estate will entails. However, the individual is confused about the potential consequences of the research, believing that the results of the study may have an impact on her care at the geriatrics clinic. Despite repeated attempts to simplify the information by breaking down sections of the informed consent document into component parts and using response cards in multiple choice format to facilitate understanding, he does not believe that the potential research participant understands that participation in this research project is completely voluntary and has no effect on her treatment in the geriatrics clinic.

Ethical Issues, Tensions, and Resources

Psychologists take reasonable steps to avoid harming others, including human research subjects (Standard 3.04, Avoiding Harm). To help avoid harmful outcomes, potential research participants must provide informed consent to research (Standard 8.02, Informed Consent to Research). Although such consent can be dispensed with under some circumstances (Standard 8.05, Dispensing With Informed Consent for Research), having cognitive deficits is not such a circumstance. Enrolling the woman in question in the research study about capacity to execute estate wills could harm her, as she cannot appreciate the consequences of participation in research, but instead believes the study will somehow affect her care in the geriatrics clinic.

The student's desire to complete his dissertation data collection by recruiting this individual and his obligation to avoid harming potential research participants (Standard 3.04, Avoiding Harm) reflects a conflict of interest (Standard 3.06, Conflict of Interest). He cannot assume a research role with patients of the clinic if doing so puts his personal needs ahead of those of potential research participants. The student must determine whether the woman in question has capacity to consent to research (Standards 3.10, Informed Consent, and Standard 8.02, Informed Consent to Research), which she does not, and then carefully and accurately document reasons for exclusion from the study (Standard 6.01, Documentation of Professional and Scientific Work and Maintenance of Records) for the IRB (Standard 8.01, Institutional Approval). Such efforts are consistent with Principle D (Justice), which provides equal access to and benefit from the contributions of psychology, by explaining why this person has been excluded. Because the potential research participant is also a patient in the geriatrics clinic, Standard 8.04 (Client/Patient, Student, and Subordinate Research Participants) regarding client/patient research participants is also pertinent to this scenario and requires consideration. This standard states that psychologists take extra precautions to ensure that declining or withdrawing from research does not result in adverse consequences for patients or clients. This is directly relevant as the potential participant in question has diminished capacity, is a client of the university geriatrics clinic, and misinterprets the research project as being a part of her direct patient care.

Preferred Course of Action

The student, however eager he may be to complete his dissertation, should exclude the woman from participation in the research project. However, if she desired help in executing an estate will, a referral to an elder law clinic or assistance from a student in either the geropsychology or financial planning clinics would be helpful. Such a referral, consistent with the principle of beneficence, would attempt to meet the woman's need with assistance in executing an important legal document.

PUBLICATION

Overview

Throughout a student or trainee's mentored experience, publication of significant intellectual work may be a goal, and beginning as early as undergraduate study, an understanding of plagiarism is necessary. Nuanced understanding of publication credit and duplicate publication of data develops with time and experience. In the beginning of graduate training, students may be included on presentations or publications of projects with lesser intellectual contribution than is required later in training, such as at the dissertation level. Modeling clear conversations regarding expectations of intellectual contribution and how this relates to order of authorship is essential for geropsychologists involved in training the next generation of scientist–practitioners. Unfortunately, except with regard to the dissertation or the extreme circumstance of having an expectation of inclusion as an author by virtue of one's position, the Ethics Code is silent on the more subtle ethical issues involved in publication credit. For example, discussions regarding order of authorship (Standard 8.12, Publication Credit) may need to be revisited periodically because intellectual contribution and effort may shift during the process of preparing the manuscript.

A typical example of the mentoring process involving an advanced trainee at the dissertation level was described in Phillips and colleagues (2004). Geropsychologists may assist or advise advanced students with the design and plan of the overall project, serve as research mentor for all phases of the project, and help conduct data analyses and interpretation of results. Following the Ethics Code and the guidelines of many universities, the student would be first author of papers based on data stemming from the dissertation except under extreme circumstances (Standard 8.12c, Publication Credit).

Kearney (2014) delineated ethical issues involving various stakeholders in the publication of student work such as master's theses and dissertations.

Such stakeholders include the student, the mentor–geropsychologist, the university, the journal editor, and the publisher. University graduate schools commonly require publication of theses and dissertations on ProQuest or other online repositories, and Kearney outlined how this may limit publication opportunities in some medical or health service journals that would consider previous online availability of a work to conflict with Standard 8.13 (Duplicate Publication of Data). For example, *The New England Journal of Medicine* precludes publication of theses or dissertations that were previously available online.

At times, delays may occur between a student's dissertation defense and publication of the work in journal article or book format. Thomas and Skinner (2012) described factors that contribute to conversion of dissertations into publications and provide a "toolkit" that facilitates this process. Contributing factors include the quality of the dissertation, consideration of the authorship or writing team, selection of the target journal or other publication outlet, and expectations about the conversion and publication process potentially through use of the toolkit. Several contextual pressures may contribute to ethical quandaries with regard to publication of a student's dissertation (Kearney, 2014; Thomas & Skinner, 2012). These include the subsequent employment setting of the student in question as well as the academic development of the mentor (i.e., tenured or on the tenure clock and therefore in greater need of publications and evidence of effective mentorship of students).

Vignette

An early career psychologist defended her dissertation on late life employment 3 years ago and subsequently accepted a job in research and development regarding employee retirement decisions for an international company. Although engaged in research daily, her work revolves around the needs of her company, and she does not have to develop her own program of research and scholarship, nor does she have pressure to publish her work in outlets outside of the company. In contrast, her dissertation chair and mentor is preparing her dossier for tenure and promotion at the university and must carefully document her scholarly publication record as well as her successful matriculation of students through the program. The two women had verbally agreed 6 months ago to submit the recent graduate's dissertation research to a respectable mid-level geriatric mental health journal and had nearly completed their work together on this project when other responsibilities arose precluding finalization and submission. The former mentor therefore submits the work with minimal additional contribution beyond their work together 6 months prior, and she lists the recent graduate as first author and herself as second author. When she submits the work, she receives an e-mail from the recent graduate describing ongoing efforts regarding publication of her dissertation with a PhD student in public health at a university in close geographic proximity to her. It is unclear to the former mentor if the recent graduate already submitted the dissertation with the newly involved student, and if her own name was on such a submission as dissertation chair.

Ethical Issues, Tensions, and Resources

Problems arose in this scenario because of the relatively informal communication style between the recent graduate and her former mentor, as well as the lengthy time between the dissertation defense and the submission of at least one manuscript stemming from the dissertation. Moreover, contextual stressors associated with their work situations add complexity and enhance the need for clear communication between the two women. As stated by Thomas and Skinner (2012), it is often beneficial for newly minted PhDs who are attempting to publish their dissertations to enlist the assistance of their former mentors in the writing and journal submission process. Certainly, mentoring a student through the dissertation process requires intellectual effort and assistance, and the mentor may well feel that she deserves authorship credit as well as the ability to report in her dossier that she successfully mentored this former student through the dissertation and publication process.

The Ethics Code is relatively silent on the more nuanced ethical issues involved in publication credit. However, in this case, issues regarding order of authorship (Standard 8.12, Publication Credit, and, potentially, Standard 8.13, Duplicate Publication of Data) could arise if both parties proceeded independently with submission and revision of this manuscript. Standard 8.12c clearly states that except in "exceptional circumstances" the student should be listed as first author of any publication stemming from his or her dissertation. The Ethics Code does not directly address whether a dissertation chair should be included as an author, directing instead that such decisions should be made based on intellectual contribution to the work. The mentor in this case submitted the manuscript with the recent graduate as first author; however, communication broke down between the two women, and their efforts seemed to evolve independently.

Preferred Course of Action

Both parties should have discussed any thoughts or plans about publication prior to either of them taking any action along those lines. Having not done that, they need to discuss any potential confusion from their prior communication about the current status of submission of the dissertation in journal article format (i.e., has there been just one submission by the mentor or has there been an additional submission by the recent graduate?). It is likely that the best avenue for such a conversation would be a real-time discussion via telephone or Skype because communication via e-mail, lacking nonverbal communication cues, can result in increased confusion. If two submissions of the dissertation have occurred to different (or the same) journals, one must be withdrawn. A clear and thorough discussion of authorship must occur prior to continuing with the submission of this dissertation in journal article format. It is likely that through clear and open communication, the issue can be resolved and both parties (and perhaps the new student working with the recent graduate) may move forward collaboratively with manuscript submission. Potentially, the mentor may also benefit from stress reduction by seeking peer support from other faculty members who are going through or have recently successfully completed the tenure and promotion process at her university.

CONCLUSION

Many geropsychologists engage in teaching, supervision, research, and mentoring activities, commonly in higher education, a VA facility, or other institutional settings. While often personally rewarding, these activities involve ethical issues that are multifaceted and thus often complex. Teaching, encouraging, and modeling high standards of ethical practice positively affects new generations of geropsychologists, whereas engaging in ethical misconduct, even when unintentional, can result in the perpetuation of inappropriate professional behavior and can discourage students, trainees, and junior colleagues from a career in a specialty that can be highly rewarding and is in great demand. Teachers, supervisors, and mentors have an expanded ethical responsibility; they are responsible for their own behavior as well as that of their students, trainees, and mentees. Thus, familiarity with relevant ethical resources and their application and a personal commitment to modeling high standards of ethical behavior take on increased importance for geropsychologists engaged in these activities.

8

SETTING-SPECIFIC ETHICAL CHALLENGES IN GEROPSYCHOLOGY

To know an object is to lead to it through a context which the world provides.

—William James

The emphases placed on different ethical issues and the ethical challenges that are confronted vary depending on the settings and contexts in which geropsychological services are provided. The nature and severity of presenting problems, degree of involvement of family members, and extent of participation of interprofessional colleagues are examples of factors that vary across settings and affect the specific services that are provided and, by extension, the relative applicability of the various ethical issues. This chapter reviews ethical issues and some common ethical challenges encountered in settings in which geropsychologists provide services. Because space limitations prevent us from covering all relevant settings and contexts, we selected settings that are either commonly encountered with older adults or are becoming increasingly important practice settings for geropsychologists: primary care, hospital units, home-based care, long-term care, forensic contexts, and hospice and palliative care.

http://dx.doi.org/10.1037/0000010-009
Ethical Practice in Geropsychology, by S. S. Bush, R. S. Allen, and V. A. Molinari
Copyright © 2017 by the American Psychological Association. All rights reserved.

PRIMARY CARE

Overview

Geropsychology practice in primary care settings is growing (Karel, Gatz, & Smyer, 2012; O'Shea Carney, Gum, & Zeiss, 2015; Scogin, Hanson, & Welsh, 2003; Scogin & Shah, 2006; Thielke, Vannoy, & Unützer, 2007; Zweig et al., 2005), resulting in greater attention to the ethics of interprofessional collaboration (Engel & Prentice, 2013). A precipitating factor for this increase is the recognition that chronic medical conditions often are accompanied by psychological disorders (Solano, Gomes, & Higginson, 2006) such as depression and anxiety (Scherrer et al., 2003). There has also been growing awareness that comorbid conditions are the rule rather than the exception with frail older adults (Schnell et al., 2012) and that "one-stop shopping" for health care provides greater ease of access (Spragins, Lorenzetti, & The Change Foundation, 2008), particularly for older adults with mental health problems.

Collaborative care is an approach in which physicians and mental health care providers work together in an organized way to manage common mental disorders and chronic disease and represents best clinical practice, particularly given the many chronic conditions experienced by many older adults (Parekh & Barton, 2010; Scherrer et al., 2003). The Interprofessional Education Collaborative (2016) provides a wealth of educational and funding resources to facilitate interprofessional primary care; however, psychology as a discipline is underrepresented. Moreover, little focus is provided on treating mental health and wellness issues among older adult patients in primary care, and older adults are less likely than young and middle-aged adults to receive treatment for mental health conditions (Karel, Gatz, & Smyer, 2012). Eighty-one percent of people with serious chronic conditions see two or more physicians each year (Anderson, Herbert, Zeffiro, & Johnson, 2010). Integrated care spans a continuum of models from colocation, in which individuals representing specific disciplines consult with each other in the same clinic space, to truly integrated interprofessional practice with shared power and decision making in interdisciplinary team meetings. An exemplary model for integrated care may be found in the Veterans Affairs (VA) medical system, which has integrated psychologists into treatment teams in primary care, home-based primary care (HBPC), community living centers (skilled nursing, rehabilitation, and palliative care), and specialized palliative care (Karel, Gatz, & Smyer, 2012).

A lack of coordination of care among health service providers has been implicated by some researchers in the underutilization of mental health services by older adults, because older adults are more likely to seek treatment in primary care settings (Institute of Medicine, 2012). Significant racial and ethnic disparities in the utilization of mental health care also exist, raising the issue of cultural competence in the provision of care. For example, African Americans' mental health utilization rate has been found to be 6.4% lower than the rate for non-Hispanic Whites (Kim et al., 2013). This disparity may reflect the problem that behavioral health integration and treatment team planning are not reimbursed commensurate with the time it takes to make a difference (Levey, Miller, & deGruy, 2012). Notably, the integration of mental health care for older adults in primary care has demonstrated consistent effectiveness in reducing negative patient outcomes (Alexopoulos et al., 2009; Hunkeler et al., 2006; Karel, Gatz, & Smyer, 2012; O'Shea Carney et al., 2015; Unützer et al., 2008).

Carpenter (2014) described an interprofessional teaching model focused on foundational competencies in interdisciplinary care for older adults. Foundational competencies include (a) understanding the theory and science of geriatric team building; (b) valuing the role that other providers play in the assessment and treatment of older clients; (c) demonstrating awareness, appreciation, and respect for team experiences, values, and discipline-specific conceptual models; and (d) understanding the importance of teamwork in geriatric settings to address the varied biopsychosocial needs of older adults. Carpenter presented data showing the teaching model's efficacy in improving preinstruction attitudes toward older adults and toward interdisciplinary care among graduate students representing multiple disciplines.

Mirroring the *Ethical Principles of Psychologists and Code of Conduct* (hereinafter, Ethics Code) (American Psychological Association [APA], 2010), but written from the perspective of nursing, Engel and Prentice (2013) contrasted the basis of Kantian ethics in which the motivation to do good is driven by the effort to do one's duty and Aristotelian ethics, which is based in a characterological desire to do good. They described the context of integrated primary care in the Canadian and U.S. health care systems. The authors highlighted differences in these systems: The Canadian system promotes the principle of justice through universality, accessibility, sustainability, and affordability of primary care to all citizens, whereas in the United States, the push toward interprofessional care stemmed from quality improvement initiatives and concerns with patient safety caused by medical errors associated with poor interprofessional communication. Engel and Prentice identified the following challenges to the provision of quality interprofessional primary care: (a) different perspectives about patient outcomes, (b) power struggles among team members, (c) lack of role clarity, (d) lack of understanding about the roles and scopes of practice of other providers, and (e) stereotyping with regard to other professions. These challenges correspond to standards in the Ethics Code, specifically Standards 2.01, Boundaries of Competence; 3.09, Cooperation with Other Professionals;

and 3.11, Psychological Services Delivered to or Through Organizations. Notably, psychology is not mentioned in Engel and Prentice's discussion of *interprofessional ethics and collaboration*, defined as essentially relational, a "shared understanding of values, beliefs and vulnerability . . . involving parity, mutual goals, shared accountability, shared resources, and voluntariness" (p. 431). Provocatively, they questioned whether collaboration can even occur; if it cannot, they asked whether it is ethical to teach and promote it: "If ethical decision making in health care implies a duty of care that resides in standards and tenets, then decision making that is highly collaborative cannot occur" (p. 432). These issues apply to the interprofessional care of older adults as illustrated in the following case example.

Vignette

A female veteran presented to the Geriatric Extended Care clinic at her local VA Medical Center in the company of her sister. The center's interdisciplinary team consisted of a geriatrician, nurse, geropsychologist, pharmacist, and social worker. The patient was a nurse in Vietnam and was 30% service-connected for posttraumatic stress disorder. She currently lived with her son in the family home. During this clinic visit, she was seen by the nurse for the taking of vital signs, the geriatrician for medical issues, the pharmacist for a review of current medications, and the social worker for a review of current benefits. She also completed a clinical interview and general cognitive and mood assessments with the geropsychologist.

The patient's sister reported to the geropsychologist that the patient had been complaining to her for some time about the living conditions with her son. She stated that the patient was worried about her son's drug problem and his spending some of her disability check on drugs in addition to managing the household. The patient's sister stated also that she would like for her sister to come and live with her to resolve some of the problematic issues arising in relation to the son.

The geropsychologist made the following observations during a clinical interview with the patient. The patient reported,

> I love my boy . . . I really do. But, you know, with his problem it's just gotten hard to live with. And I know he takes care of me and loves me. But I know what he does with some of the money.

When asked about her preferred living situation, the patient stated that she wanted to live with her sister because "I know she will take care of me and just focus on me. Take care of me." On a cognitive screening evaluation the patient obtained a score of 19, which is in the range typically associated with dementia (Fernandez-Ballesteros, Marquez-Gonzalez, & Santacreu,

2014; Lengenfelder & DeLuca, 2005). Her scores on screening measures of depression and anxiety were unremarkable.

In addition to gathering information about the patient's current health status, at the interdisciplinary team meeting the geriatrician asked for the opinions of the team regarding the patient's desire to live with her sister. Members of the team were in general agreement that the two women should live together. Individuals of different disciplines varied, however, on their assessment of the patient's capacity to make decisions and on whether to consider reporting the issue to Adult Protective Services as a possible case of financial abuse.

Ethical Decision-Making Process

The sequence of ethical decision-making questions and steps in Exhibits 3.1 and 3.2 provides a structured approach to addressing ethical challenges. Asking oneself the questions and following the steps for each case is likely to help achieve good outcomes.

Ethical and Legal Issues

Standards 2.01, Boundaries of Competence; 3.09, Cooperation with Other Professionals; and 3.11, Psychological Services Delivered to or Through Organizations, are relevant (APA, 2010). In interdisciplinary teams, it is important to define roles and expectations to foster effective communication. The geropsychologist must work with other team members to communicate that although the patient scored in the dementia range on a cognitive screening exam, that fact alone does not negate her ability to state a valid preference regarding with whom she wants to live. Therefore, the geropsychologist must navigate boundaries of competence within the interprofessional team and cooperate with other team members in an effective manner (O'Shea Carney et al., 2015). As the geriatric extended care clinic at the treatment facility has a structured hierarchy of practice, the geropsychologist was mindful that services are provided as a part of this clinic and that, likely as an example of psychological services delivered to or through organizations, the geriatrician would be tasked with making the final decision as to whether to report the case to Adult Protective Services.

Ethical and Legal Tensions

Tensions may have arisen in relation to differing opinions on reporting potential financial abuse of the patient by her son. Different professions hold different values in relation to the principles of respect for autonomy and beneficence, so the relative weight of emphasis on the patient's ability to competently state a wish for her living situation also may have varied. The leadership of the geriatrician during the interdisciplinary team meeting, however, represents a relative strength of this team in the ethics of interprofessional primary care. In other words, the geriatrician illustrated collaborative leadership by proactively gathering all of the team members into the care planning meeting and listening to each professional's perspective on the case. This facilitates open communication and shared and informed decision making.

Preferred Course of Action

The likely preferred course of action would be for a mental health professional such as the geropsychologist on the team to work with the patient and the patient's sister on enacting the patient's preferred living situation. Additionally, developing a consensus and making a decision about whether to report potential financial abuse regarding the patient's VA disability check would be necessary for the interprofessional team members to maintain and, perhaps, enhance their collaborative relationships. By training, geropsychologists are well-prepared to foster collaborative group dynamics and provide education about biopsychosocial issues. Within this context, the geropsychologist would be well-prepared to lead a group discussion about the decision to report the situation to Adult Protective Services.

HOSPITAL UNITS

Overview

Older adults, compared with younger populations, have a higher incidence of significant medical problems. As a result, the rates of hospitalization are higher for older adults (Centers for Disease Control and Prevention, 2010). Although older adults comprised only 12% of the U.S. population in 2003, they accounted for more than 33% of all hospital admissions (Russo & Elixhauser, 2006). Geropsychologists working in hospital settings provide a variety of assessment, treatment, and educational services that benefit older adults and their families. Assessment services cover a wide range of activities, including (a) determinations of cognitive capacity to consent to surgery or other medical procedures or to make decisions regarding discharge and medications; (b) cognitive evaluations for diagnostic purposes, such as to clarify the presence and nature of dementias or delirium; and (c) clarification of emotional states, pain, behavioral challenges, personality traits, and the interaction of emotional and physical symptoms as commonly encountered in both established medical illnesses and somatic symptom disorders. Identification of suicidal thoughts and dangerousness to others is frequently a focus of assessments. Assessment measures are also commonly used to establish the evidence base for treatment services or quality improvement, such as through brief, serial assessments of emotional symptoms.

Psychological treatment services provided to older adults on hospital units often address adjustment to illness, injury, or functional changes; pain management; or sleep disorders. Treatment may be provided in individual, group, or family therapy formats. Educational services commonly target psychological factors contributing to medical illness with the intent of establishing biopsychosocial lifestyle changes to improve health and functioning. Both patients and their family members are often recipients of educational services.

Geropsychological services provided in acute hospital settings are unique in many ways because of the (a) severity of patient injury or illness, (b) involvement of numerous other professionals and support staff, (c) relatively brief duration of stay, and (d) often loud and intrusive nature of the environment. The uniqueness of the setting provides clinical opportunities and challenges for geropsychologists, often with corresponding ethical challenges. Geropsychologists who are aware of common ethical challenges can often develop strategies to avoid ethical dilemmas and prepare to address these challenges when they arise.

Vignette

A 66-year-old woman is admitted to an oncology service with recently diagnosed Stage IVA lung cancer. She begins receiving radiation treatments and chemotherapy. She also has a morphine drip and is receiving supplemental oxygen. She is very frightened and upset and accepts the case manager's offer to call in a psychologist to talk with her. The psychologist, however, is completely booked with clinical, administrative, and supervisory responsibilities for that day and the next, so he decides he will see the patient first thing on her third day in the hospital. When he gets to her room on the date he had in mind, she is out of the room for radiation treatment. He decides to check back at the end of the day. When he goes back, she is very tired and seems a bit confused, and her family is sitting with her. He informs them that he will return the following day. He writes a progress note in the patient's chart questioning whether she is appropriate for psychotherapy at this time, given her confusion, and stating that she seems to have adequate support from family members for the time being. He notes his intention to return the following day. He is unable to visit her the next morning because of other commitments, so he plans to return in the early afternoon, when he knows she is available. However, just prior to the time that he planned to see her, he is called by his supervisor and informed that an anticipated site visit by the Joint Commission is underway and that his presence is required in the supervisor's office. He attempts to explain the scheduling issue, but his supervisor seems frazzled and focused only on the Joint Commission. The psychologist decides that he will definitely see the patient the following day. When he arrives at her room the following afternoon, he learns that she has been discharged to a palliative care unit in a long-term care facility. He is very disappointed that he never had a chance to spend time with her.

Ethical Issues, Tensions, and Resources

The geropsychologist has multiple demands on his time in a very busy hospital setting. Assessment and treatment of anxiety and depression in patients with cancer are consistent with professional guidelines, which states,

> Although clinicians may not be able to prevent some of the chronic or late medical effects of cancer, they have a vital role in mitigating the negative emotional and behavioral sequelae. Recognizing and treating effectively those who manifest symptoms of anxiety or depression will reduce the human cost of cancer. (Andersen et al., 2014, p. 1605)

Whereas caring for patients is his priority (Principle A: Beneficence and Nonmaleficence), the psychologist cannot simply abandon his other responsibilities (Principle B: Fidelity and Responsibility). The decisions he made in this case were not in the patient's best interests, and they reflected poorly on psychology within the treatment team, but they were required in order for the psychology service and his role in it to remain viable overall. When he realized that he would not be able to see this distressed patient right away, psychologist could have tried to refer her to another mental health professional (e.g., the team social worker or psychiatrist) or a trainee (Standard 3.09, Cooperation with Other Professionals). Following her discharge, he could ask the case manager, or take the initiative himself, to contact the long-term care facility to make sure the new treatment team is aware of the need for the patient to receive mental health services as soon as possible.

Professional tensions resulting from many, perhaps too many, responsibilities led to an ethical tension between the principles of beneficence and responsibility. Because he had responsibilities to the patient and treatment team, as well as to his trainees, the psychology department, and the institution, he was forced to prioritize his efforts.

The Ethics Code (APA, 2010) describes the relevant principles and standards; however, the ability to work out the logistics so that the principles of beneficence and responsibility can both be satisfied in such a demanding setting would likely require input from an experienced colleague. The geropsychologist's supervisor may be an excellent resource for this purpose (but only after the Joint Commission leaves). In the interim, a more senior psychologist on staff in the department or a trusted colleague practicing somewhere else could provide more immediate recommendations for managing the situation. Understanding that the average hospital length of stay for persons age 65 and older is 5.5 days (Centers for Disease Control and Prevention, 2010) may help the geropsychologist establish appropriate professional priorities.

Preferred Course of Action

The geropsychologist had a number of options at his disposal but did not appear to know that he needed them until it was too late. At each decision point, it seemed to him that he would be able to meet with the patient in a reasonable time frame. In retrospect, among his many options, he could have (a) asked the case manager to refer the patient to another mental health professional; (b) determined when the patient was scheduled to be available and awake, given her various treatments and response to them, and rearranged his schedule, if possible, so that their schedules would coincide for a brief period; (c) perhaps met with her while she was receiving one of her treatments; or (d) asked a trainee to see her or used the supervision time for them both to see her. Having a plan or policy in place that described steps to take when an urgent referral is received but there is no time to meet with the patient could have helped satisfy the needs of all parties. Although such a plan was not developed prospectively, creating one after the fact could promote high standards of ethical practice in the future.

HOME-BASED CARE

Overview

The current model of health care involves a combination of office-based primary care, specialist consultations, hospital admission, brief rehabilitation stays, and long-term institutional care. Many older adults are unable to pursue medical or mental health care in the community setting of their choice. Approximately 12 million Americans receive in-home services each year (National Association for Home Care & Hospice, 2015). Medical problems, functional limitations, lack of access to transportation, cost containment, and changing values that emphasize living and dying at home are among the many reasons for the growing popularity of home-based care. According to National Association for Home Care & Hospice, in 2009 it cost Medicare nearly $6,200 per day for a typical hospital stay and $622 per day for a typical nursing home stay, whereas home care cost just $135 per visit. Seegert (2013), of the Association of Health Care Journalists, reported that the demand for home-based services is expected to continue rising.

> Home-based primary care (HBPC) interventions have roots in the house call and community health outreach of the past. Today, HBPC is a model that combines home-based care for medical needs with intense

management, care coordination, as well as long-term services and supports (LTSS) when needed. (U.S. Department of Health and Human Services, Agency for Healthcare Research and Quality, 2014)

Home-based primary care, formerly called *hospital-based home care*, was developed by the VA in the early 1970s. Although elements vary across sites, current HBPC programs consist of a physician-supervised interdisciplinary team that provides care in the home to veterans with complex needs for whom functional limitations render clinic-based care difficult to obtain or ineffective.

The HBPC patients are among the sickest in the VA health care system, averaging 19 clinical diagnoses and 15 medications (Egan, 2012). The average age of veterans receiving HBPC is 76.5 years, and 96% are male, which is not unexpected given the traditionally higher proportion of males in the military (Egan, 2012). A significant percentage of veterans receiving HBPC services have cognitive or psychological problems: depression (44%), dementia (33%), substance abuse (29%), and schizophrenia (20%). Not listed are the many other psychological problems that veterans with chronic health conditions and functional limitations commonly experience, such as adjustment disorders, anxiety disorders, and posttraumatic stress disorder. High rates of psychiatric disorders have also been found in civilian geriatric home care patients (Davitt & Gellis, 2011; Zeltzer & Kohn, 2006). Thus, the need for psychological services in this population is great, and geropsychologists are well-positioned to provide valuable care to patients in their homes.

The potential benefits of HBPC are many (see Exhibit 8.1). Despite the potential advantages of HBPC, "uncertainties remain about potential harms, unintended consequences, costs, and sustainability of this model of care. In some cases, evaluations and research studies have contributed to, rather than

EXHIBIT 8.1
Advantages of Home-Based Primary Care

- Increased access to care for people who have difficulty traveling to outpatient medical offices
- Safer care for people for whom going to a medical office or hospital is contra-indicated, such as those particularly vulnerable to infections or those with cognitive deficits who may become more confused and/or agitated
- Better understanding of patients' environments, needs, and constraints that can improve care and ultimately outcomes
- Decreased hospitalizations and urgent care use when acute incidents are prevented or addressed in the home
- Potential for prevention or slowing of functional and cognitive decline
- Better support for and reduced burden on family caregivers
- Cost savings

Note. Data from U.S. Department of Health and Human Services, Agency for Healthcare Research and Quality (2014) and the National Association for Home Care and Hospice (2010).

resolved, this uncertainty" (U.S. Department of Health and Human Services, Agency for Healthcare Research and Quality, 2014). Because of considerable methodological differences among studies of HBPC, "there remain questions about which outcomes best match the different goals of different versions of HBPC and which outcomes are most important to different patients" (U.S. Department of Health and Human Services, Agency for Healthcare Research and Quality, 2014).

The evolution of the VA model has included more mental health services and improved collaboration with other services. The model of integrated mental health care in HBPC is informed by evidence-based models of geriatric mental health care delivery (Gordon & Karel, 2014). Care teams currently consist of physicians, medical directors, nurses, social workers, dieticians, psychologists, pharmacists, and rehabilitative therapists who coordinate with one another, the patient, and the patient's family members when applicable and provide referrals for additional services as needed (Egan, 2012; U.S. Department of Health and Human Services, Agency for Healthcare Research and Quality, 2014; U.S. Department of Veterans Affairs, 2015). Gordon and Karel (2014) observed,

> In HBPC, the mental health provider not only provides specialized assessment and intervention services, but, at the foundation of HBPC care, partners with the team in providing interdisciplinary, patient-centered, and collaborative care for all enrolled veterans. The mental health provider works with the team, through care management and stepped care approaches, to determine which veterans would benefit from specialized mental health services. In those cases, the mental health provider evaluates the veteran and provides recommendations to the team and behavioral/mental health interventions as indicated. (p. 129)

Yang, Garis, Jackson, and McClure (2009) discussed three specific ethical issues often encountered when conducting in-home therapy: confidentiality threats, multiple relationships, and "complicated" informed consent. Regarding confidentiality, curious neighbors or even overlapping health care professionals serving the client may want to know why the geropsychologist is coming to visit the client. Having a predetermined plan in place developed early in treatment may help the client be comfortable with what is revealed to these concerned others and may preserve the client's autonomous right not to disclose personal information.

Regarding the multiple relationships that are confronted in in-home therapy, geropsychologists may face situations in which they feel an urge to act outside of their role. For example, the geropsychologist may encounter hungry clients with no food in the house or hazardous conditions that may need immediate solutions. Should the professional fix a meal or move the obstruction out of the way, tasks that some in-home clients may be unable to perform without help? Behaving within a rigid professional role in such cases for fear of "crossing boundaries" may not be in the best interests of the client who needs immediate attention, may not be consistent with the beneficence principle, and may adversely affect rapport. However, reporting to Adult Protective Services, coordinating a comprehensive action plan to remedy the situation, or recommending a higher level of care than community care may not do justice to the principle of respect for autonomy if done in a hasty manner.

Regarding informed consent, geropsychologists conducting in-home visits may arrive at a home at the assigned time, but the client may not answer the door even though the geropsychologist can see through the window that the person is indeed at home. Working under the principle of beneficence by knocking loudly until the client opens the door may clarify the situation and allow the geropsychologist to make a pitch for what additional mental health services can offer, but may not reflect respect for autonomy, which would afford the client the ability to decline the visit. Finally, visiting clients in unsafe neighborhoods where they may possess firearms pits the beneficent need to help others with the equally valid concern for one's own personal safety (Yang et al., 2009).

A variation of HBPC that uses telecommunication technology in the delivery of mental health (referred to as *telemental health*) provides expanded access to psychological services. Clinical video technology allows psychologists to assess patients from remote locations, which is particularly advantageous for patients, many of whom are older adults and cannot travel long distances to medical centers. As with HBPC, the use of telemental health, including clinical video technology, has been pioneered by the VA. The three primary areas in which assessment of veterans occurs via telemental health technology are neuropsychological testing, suicide assessment, and clinical outcome assessment (Yoder & Turner, 2014). Although still developing and not without its limitations, expanded clinical use of this technology is expected, and the use of telemental health technology "in patients' homes and eventually mobile devices will likely become commonplace" (Yoder & Turner, 2014, p. 165).

Innovative approaches to patient care are accompanied by ethical issues that must be considered and addressed in order for the novel system to become and remain viable. Geropsychologists who are aware of and appropriately address the ethical issues serve an important function in the assessment and treatment of older adults in unique contexts.

Vignette

A geropsychologist, working as part of a VA HBPC team, evaluates an 88-year-old widowed African American veteran in his home. Although the veteran does not seem to have problems with orientation, memory, or other cognitive abilities during the clinical interview, the geropsychologist administers the Mini-Mental State Examination (MMSE) as she routinely does with new patients. During the registration (naming and learning three objects) portion of the MMSE, the patient's son walks into the home, says hello to everyone, and then goes into a different room. During the attention and calculation portion of the exam, the phone begins ringing until the patient's son answers it in another room. With a total score of 21 on the MMSE and functional limitations, the geropsychologist diagnoses the veteran as having major neurocognitive disorder and recommends to the HBPC team that the veteran be sent to a neurologist for an MRI of the brain and possibly started on a trial of an acetylcholinesterase inhibitor.

Ethical Issues, Tensions, and Resources

The potential for multiple and unexpected distractions exists when providing psychological services in patients' homes. Geropsychologists strive to anticipate distractions and to manage the environment to the extent possible so that the results of the evaluation will be a valid reflection of the patient's cognitive and emotional functioning; such efforts are needed for competent practice in this subspecialty (Standard 2.01, Boundaries of Competence). The geropsychologist was unable to control the environment enough to obtain valid cognitive test results. Although including an objective measure of cognition was an attempt to use empirical evidence to support clinical decision making (Standard 2.04, Bases for Scientific and Professional Judgments; Standard 9.01, Bases for Assessments), misinterpreting invalid results has the potential to be more harmful than beneficial and is therefore inconsistent with Principle A (Beneficence and Nonmaleficence) and reinforces concerns about the geropsychologist's professional competence. Although the geropsychologist's race and cultural background are not described, the issue of cultural competence is also essential to consider when evaluating ethnic minority patients.

When interpreting assessment results, psychologists need to

> take into account . . . the various test factors, test-taking abilities and other characteristics of the person being assessed, such as situational, personal, linguistic and cultural differences, that might affect psychologists' judgments or reduce the accuracy of their interpretations. They indicate any significant limitations of their interpretations. (Standard 9.06, Interpreting Assessment Results)

This geropsychologist did not take into account the situational or cultural influences or indicate any limitations of her interpretations. Because the test results could not be considered valid, questions about which norms were used or the possible impact of quality of education or cultural differences on test performance did not need to be raised. The geropsychologist's decisions and actions may have resulted in misdiagnosis and inappropriate recommendations.

In her efforts to make sound clinical decisions that promote the patient's well-being (beneficence), the geropsychologist needed to determine whether to administer any psychometric measure in this context and, if so, how to reduce the possibility or impact of environmental distractions and how to interpret the results if such distractions occur despite efforts to avoid them. Relying on the clinical interview, behavioral observations, and medical records may have been adequate to obtain the needed information without risking arriving at potentially harmful conclusions as a result of invalid inferences from inadequate testing procedures (nonmaleficence).

The geropsychologist in this case seems unaware that any of her actions reflect functional incompetence or that her decisions should be questioned or could have ethical implications. The Ethics Code (APA, 2010) is a primary resource for the ethical issues needed to help determine what could be done in the future to help reduce the likelihood of misdiagnosis and inappropriate recommendations in such situations, as well as how to address the problem if a colleague should question the diagnosis or recommendations. Scholarly publications also provide valuable perspectives and recommendations for promoting good clinical and ethical practice when evaluating racially and culturally diverse older adults (e.g., Byrd & Manly, 2012; Rivera Mindt, Arentoft, Coulehan, & Byrd, 2013) and deciding whether the advantages of using a screening measure outweigh the disadvantages (Lengenfelder & DeLuca, 2005).

Preferred Course of Action

During the early to middle stages of the process of administering the test when multiple distractions occurred, the geropsychologist should have immediately understood that the results would not be a valid representation of the patient's true cognitive abilities. Test administration should have been discontinued, and no attempt to interpret the results should have been made. If, after considering the other sources of information, the geropsychologist believed that cognitive testing would be informative, a plan could have been established to perform the testing under better circumstances (e.g., an office or better controlled home environment) or a referral to a neuropsychologist could have been made. Given that the geropsychologist administered and interpreted the entire MMSE despite the distractions, she should have described the likely impact of the distractions on the results and limited her diagnostic conclusions and recommendations accordingly. The geropsychologist may also have been able to interview the patient's son after he arrived to gather collateral information, but there was no indication that she did so.

LONG-TERM CARE

Overview

Long-term care, which addresses the needs of frail, cognitively compromised, and vulnerable elders who desire to "age in place" despite major functional impairments, is rife with ethical dilemmas. This section focuses on institutional long-term care, particularly assisted living facilities and nursing homes, but many of the issues and ethical principles described in the context of these settings are generalizable to community long-term care.

As has long been noted, nursing homes resemble the old state psychiatric hospitals in the wide prevalence of mental health conditions (Burns et al., 1993). Approximately 50% of the residents have dementia (Magaziner et al., 2000), and at least half of these will exhibit behavioral difficulties. Furthermore, approximately 10% of the residents have serious mental illness (Becker & Mehra, 2010). Many other residents are reeling from the psychological sequelae of the medical conditions that decreased their functional status, thereby reducing capacity for independent living, necessitating moving away from their homes and living in an institutional setting. Those with personality disorders may wreak havoc in institutional settings and present a unique set of clinical and ethical challenges when an already fragile social support system is further weakened. These individuals may be ill-equipped to adapt to an unfamiliar communal living situation as a result of lifelong poor coping mechanisms and exaggerated, rigid personality traits (Molinari, 1999). The ability of nursing homes to be able to train their staff to manage such an array of psychiatric problems, in addition to the myriad comorbid medical conditions that need attention, remains an unsettled question.

Psychologists must do what they can in this high-need but low-resourced environment of care. As early as 1987, the Omnibus Budget Reconciliation Act (OBRA) promoted nonpsychopharmacological treatments for those with mental health problems and instituted strict guidelines regarding the use of antipsychotic medications and restraints for the behavior problems of nursing home residents, yet the full promise of OBRA has not been realized. In 1998, a group of psychologists working in long-term care published the *Standards for Psychological Services in Long Term Care Facilities* (Lichtenberg et al., 1998). These standards outlined some of the formidable challenges that psychologists face when they provide assessment and intervention services in long-term care, and they posited a series of ethical guidelines to inform practice in these settings, focusing on informed consent, confidentiality, and privacy issues.

With so many psychologically and cognitively impaired older adults residing in these long-term care settings, it is no wonder that ethical issues involving informed consent come into play early on as the psychologist struggles with concerns regarding the basics of mental health service provision. If a gero-psychologist is called in by a nursing home administrator who says the family will pay to treat a relative who is exhibiting periodic aggression toward nursing aides, it must first be decided who the client is. Is it the nursing home, which is concerned about the well-being of the staff? Is it the family who is footing the bill? Or is it the client who is receiving treatment? Principle A (Beneficence and Nonmaleficence) makes it clear that regardless of who is paying for services, and with the understanding that ethical obligations are owed to all involved parties, the psychologist owes top fealty to the client being served and should advocate for the client's best interests (Standards 3.07, Third-Party Requests for Services, and 3.11, Psychological Services Delivered to or Through Organizations). Person-centered care is of most importance but, to sustain optimal treatment, the facility and family often must be kept informed as well, particularly when a behavioral treatment plan is implemented by the nursing home staff and the finances are managed by a family conservator as a result of adjudicated incompetence of the resident. Given that the relationship between the psychologist provider, client, family, and nursing home is often in flux, the psychologist regularly monitors the informed consent status of the resident (Standards 3.10, Informed Consent, and 10.01, Informed Consent to Therapy) to assure that the client is always apprised and, to the extent possible, assents to treatment even if cognitively and legally unable to grant true legal consent. The concept of "geriatric assent" extends Principle A (Beneficence and Nonmaleficence), promoting an active partnership between the health care team and cognitively impaired client to maximize even an incapacitated older adult's input into decision making. The geropsychologist should be actively engaged in a process that involves identifying the patient's long-standing values, determining whether the treatment plan has a suitable balance of safety and independence in concordance with the patient's preferences, and safeguarding the residual autonomy of the patient, while in the course reflecting and fostering professional virtues (Coverdale, McCullough, Molinari, & Workman, 2006).

A related issue to informed consent is that of confidentiality (Standard 4: Privacy and Confidentiality). Although the policies of the Health Insurance Portability and Accountability Act of 1996 are often implemented in ways that are unnecessarily burdensome, protecting the confidential information of cognitively intact older adults treated in outpatient settings is frequently a straightforward matter. Confidentiality rights, with limitations imposed by law, allow the competent patient to be the one to determine which information is shared with the geropsychologist, family members, and other health care providers. However, in long-term care settings where a team of staff and consulting professionals are providing services to a number of residents, the geropsychologist's confidentiality responsibilities and requirements can become confusing. How and with whom information is shared (Standard 3.09, Cooperation with Other Professionals)? When the nursing home psychologist conducts an evaluation and writes a report that is placed in a resident's chart, all health care professionals are privy to the information because the institutional consent process obviates the need for each professional to garner individual consent. With the Patient Protection and Affordable Care Act (ACA; 2010) promotion of integrated care, an evidence-based practice that has been shown to promote better outcomes for older adults (Areán & Gum, 2013; Zeiss & Steffen, 1996), and confidentiality issues have gained more prominence especially as electronic health care records become a vehicle to promote interdisciplinary teamwork. Consistent with Principle B (Fidelity and Responsibility), a psychologist working in long-term care settings must present essential data about the client in a clear way without inclusion of personally interesting yet irrelevant details so as to convey the core findings and prevent misinterpretation. This is especially true when the client is revealing information about the facility or family members that can be potentially embarrassing.

Personal privacy issues (Standard 4.04, Minimizing Intrusions on Privacy) are endemic in long-term care settings and encompass very practical concerns over how to maintain a safe and secure dyadic therapeutic relationship. In outpatient settings, privacy is promoted when office doors are closed to prevent minimal outside intrusions. In the long-term care setting, rooms with two or more beds are the rule rather than the exception, and the psychologist is often faced with bedridden residents and roommates, blaring overhead announcements, confused residents, unlockable doors, rehabilitation appointments taking precedence over psychotherapeutic schedules, and medical necessities preempting the intimacy of the provider-therapist encounter. Psychologists working in these settings must make the best of a bad situation, rather than despairing of being able to adhere faithfully to the standard of privacy. Principle D (Justice) supports the idea of making good-faith planning efforts to do the best one can to offer services in such difficult circumstances lest underprivileged clients remain short-changed by an institutional system of care. Psychologists may conduct valid evaluations and effective psychotherapy in a thoughtful and respectful way, perhaps by scheduling sessions at those times when the roommate is away at a rehabilitation session (if the patient is bedridden), or finding a quiet place away from loud televisions and other residents (if the patient can walk or use a wheelchair). Informing unit staff that psychological services are about to be provided, placing a "do not disturb" sign on the door, and pulling curtains around the patient's bed can also promote privacy. The availability of private offices for such treatment may reflect the value that a long-term care setting assigns mental health interventions, and staff consultation and advocacy to educate the administration regarding the needs of psychological consultants may be in order.

A related standard that should be highlighted is practicing within one's scope of competence (Standard 2.01, Boundaries of Competence). Geropsychology has achieved the milestones of being designated as a specialty by both APA and the American Board of Professional Psychology because there is now a core distinct body of knowledge; specific training models to convey this knowledge; and well-defined geropsychology competencies in assessment, intervention, and consultation to apply this knowledge. Psychologists who practice in long-term care settings are often considered subspecialists within geropsychology, and there is a growing body of empirical knowledge reflecting unique competencies in this subspecialty. Because there are few graduate programs with tracks in geropsychology, many psychologists, especially those who graduated more than a decade ago, may not be aware of these developments in the applied aging arena. They may not recognize that optimal treatment in long-term care settings requires that providers have a unique skill set that integrates generalist psychological skills with the knowledge base of geropsychology (with some rehabilitation psychology, health psychology, and palliative care content) and its burgeoning applied evidence base within long-term care. Fortunately, there is a large volume of educational resources accessible to postlicensure psychologists, which may assist them in evaluating (Karel, Gatz, & Smyer, 2012) and upgrading their attitudes, knowledge, and skills so that they are able to work within their scope of practice in an area that sorely needs qualified geropsychologists (Karel, Molinari, Emery-Tiburcio, & Knight, 2015). To maintain one's integrity (Principle C), one must have the credentials to substantiate one's presentation as a competent professional who is able to deliver effective services yielding positive outcomes. To adhere to Principle D (Justice), psychologists must exercise reasonable judgment and take precautions to ensure that their potential biases, the boundaries of their competence, and the limitations of their expertise do not lead to or condone inferior practices with long-term care residents. Finally, to observe Principle E (Respect for People's Rights and Dignity), geropsychologists must walk a fine line between providing mental health services within a hierarchically structured, medicalized environment and advocating for culture change and a humanistic cast to service delivery.

Vignette

An 85-year-old, White male resident has become increasingly irritable with the nursing home staff, culminating in his slapping one of the nursing aides yesterday morning after she tried to bathe him. The nursing home contacted his daughter and told her that if this behavior continued, he would either be put on psychiatric medications to "calm him down," hospitalized to get the behavior under control, or transferred from the nursing home to one that had a specialized behavioral unit.

The resident has lived in the nursing home for 3 years, after a stroke left him paralyzed on the left side and unable to manage living independently. He had done well in rehabilitation and was able to begin speaking again with just some minor residual impairment, but his cognition appears to have gotten worse over the last few months. Two weeks ago his beloved sister died; since that time he has stayed in his room, has not engaged in his typical activities, has been eating less, has been exhibiting poor grooming, and has refused to bathe. His daughter contacted the geropsychologist to assist her in dealing with the problem behavior. The daughter tells the geropsychologist that she has taken over her father's legal and financial affairs by serving as his power of attorney, although she has never been officially appointed his legal guardian.

Before meeting with the resident and commencing services, the geropsychologist discusses payment for her services with the resident's daughter and the nursing home, identifies the resident as the individual to whom she owes primary allegiance, and explains that they will be kept informed of treatment progress to the extent that the resident allows.

The geropsychologist meets with the resident in his room, and on the basis of a brief conversation the resident agrees to allow information to be shared with his daughter and the nursing home medical staff, but it is unclear whether he is currently competent to consent to treatment. The geropsychologist develops good rapport with the resident, who agrees to undergo a formal evaluation even though he voices uncertainty about how he will pay for it. When the geropsychologist returns the next day to conduct the evaluation, she realizes that there is no private office available for an assessment. To make matters worse, the resident does not want to leave his bed, and his roommate is watching television. The geropsychologist requests that the roommate turn the television's volume down, pulls the curtain around the resident's bedside, and proceeds to administer some cognitive and mood tests in a muted but comprehensible voice.

Although the assessment session did not meet perfect administration standards, the geropsychologist believes that the test results are valid and reflective of mild cognitive impairment (but not serious enough to warrant a capacity evaluation) and of severe depression related to the death of his sister. During the interview that preceded the testing, the resident mentions that the new nursing aide who has been assigned him is a bit rough with him and does not make his bath as comfortable as the previous nursing assistant. On the day of the slapping incident, the resident said the aide was in a bad mood and didn't check the temperature of the bath water. However, the resident said that he didn't want the aide to get into trouble and make the aide mad at him, so he didn't want this information to be put in his record.

The geropsychologist said she understood his concerns but that she would need to convey this information to the administration so that the aide could be reassigned to prevent an escalation of this behavior and perhaps an even more negative outcome necessitating a report to Adult Protective Services.

The geropsychologist tells the resident that on the basis of his score on the mood test, she recommended a course of psychotherapy for him and that she would work with the director of nursing to secure a private room where they could talk. The geropsychologist also asks the resident what information he does not want charted in his progress notes and says that she would abide by his wishes except for those times she felt it was essential that the staff receive this information. Under those circumstances, she says she would apprise him of the exception and seek to make him feel comfortable with the information she included in his chart.

Ethical Issues, Tensions, and Resources

A major tension is how a geropsychologist can deliver services in an ethical manner within a geriatric setting that is not well-suited to allow an individual to maintain personal privacy and to keep information confidential (Standard 4: Privacy and Confidentiality). Another consideration is how to provide beneficial services (Principle A, Beneficence and Nonmaleficence) and safeguard the interests of an older adult client while at the same time being beholden to the client's family for payment (Standard 3.10, Informed Consent; Principle B: Responsibility and Fidelity). A final issue relates to how one can honor a client's concerns regarding not wanting to lodge a complaint against a formal caregiver while at the same time discharging one's duty by adhering to the state statutes regarding elder abuse. When considering how to resolve the ethical challenges, the geropsychologist considers a variety of professional resources, including the Ethics Code, other guidelines (e.g., *Guidelines for Psychological Practice With Older Adults*, APA, 2014c), and scholarly publications related to standards of practice in long-term care settings (Lichtenberg et al., 1998; Rosowsky, Casciani, & Arnold, 2008).

Regarding delivering services in a long-term care setting, the choice is either to modify what one can or else maintain the status quo and not provide any services (Principle D: Justice). On the one hand, even if the nursing home makes available a private room for psychologist visits, other residents may still intuit that the person is seeing a health professional and perhaps even react negatively. On the other hand, this resident is in need of psychological services and should be accorded them in the best manner consistent with the setting in which the person resides. Likewise, the geropsychologist must attempt to adhere to confidentiality of personal information while at the same time recognizing the rights of family members to obtain information about the course of treatment so as to feel comfortable with continuing payment for necessary services. In these regards, the limits of a geropsychologist's flexibility and tolerance for ambiguity regarding confidentiality of information (Standard 4.01, Maintaining Confidentiality) and personal privacy (Standard 4.04, Minimizing Intrusions on Privacy) concerns must be guided by a duty to act in the best interests of the client (Principle A: Beneficence and Nonmaleficence). However, the geropsychologist must strictly adhere to the statutes of the jurisdiction regarding the possibility of elder abuse, and in so doing must find a way to protect the client from any form of retaliation and process any feelings of guilt if the caregiver continues to provide services in a substandard manner.

Standard 2.01c, Competence, states: "Psychologists planning to provide services, teach or conduct research involving populations, areas, techniques or technologies new to them undertake relevant education, training, supervised experience, consultation or study." Based on this standard, the clinician's identity as a geropsychologist is based on her coursework in aging at the graduate level and supervised geriatric rotations at the internship and postdoctoral levels. To develop and maintain her competence to practice in nursing homes (Standard 2.03, Maintaining Competence), she has earned a large number of continuing education credits by attending presentations on providing psychological services in long-term care settings, and she is a member of a professional organization, Psychologists in Long Term Care, comprising psychologists who provide services in long-term care settings.

Preferred Course of Action

The geropsychologist did her best to obtain a valid assessment of the resident's cognitive decision-making capacity, respecting his right to privacy and confidentiality, despite the environmental threats to privacy, confidentiality, and optimal testing conditions. Striving to modify environmental conditions to maximize patient care in settings in which the geropsychologist's control over the environment is limited is often the best that can be done. Working with nursing staff to reduce intrusions, and obtaining the resident's informed consent or assent to undergo an evaluation under such conditions, promotes good patient care.

Regarding fees and payment responsibilities and arrangements, the geropsychologist should have clarified these issues with all involved parties before providing services, unless she was willing to waive her fee if the resident, his insurance carrier, the institution, or the patient's daughter were unable or unwilling to pay for the services after they had been provided. While occasional pro bono services are consistent with high standards of ethical practice, it is unrealistic to expect clinicians to provide free services on a regular basis.

Additionally, expectations about whether or to what extent the party paying for the service expects or needs to receive the results should be covered. While such arrangements are commonly agreed upon by all parties, exceptions exist, requiring geropsychologists to clarify the issues before proceeding with assessment or treatment services.

The issue of reporting alleged mistreatment by caregivers can be more complex than it might seem on the surface. For example, for residents who have cognitive or serious psychiatric disorders, the accuracy of the alleged mistreatment must be considered. Nevertheless, unless strong evidence exists to doubt the accuracy of the resident's report, such poor caregiver behavior must be taken very seriously, and addressing it must be a priority. Geropsychologists' clinical skills are often put to excellent use in such situations in their efforts to help residents understand that their well-being is the primary consideration and that every reasonable effort will be made to ensure that quality nursing care is maintained or improved and that no retaliation of any kind will be forthcoming. The geropsychologist will then need to follow institutional and jurisdictional reporting requirements, typically first by meeting with the director of nursing and the facility's administrator to plan a remedial course of action.

FORENSIC CONTEXTS

Overview

Geropsychologists frequently encounter assessment questions and referrals regarding the capacity of an older adult to perform activities necessary for autonomous and independent living, including but not limited to managing medications or finances, driving, maintaining a household, or making decisions about medical care or future distribution of assets. Three general areas of professional ethics are particularly important within this area of practice: competence, human relations, and privacy or confidentiality.

Over the past four decades, perhaps the most explosive growth in knowledge pertinent to civil forensic issues encountered by geropsychologists is work regarding assessment of and intervention with older adults with diminished capacity (American Bar Association/APA Assessment of Capacity in Older Adults Project Working Group, 2008; Moye, Marson, & Edelstein, 2013). Moye et al. (2013) described six areas of future growth in research and practice regarding civil capacity evaluations: (a) linking capacity research to neuroscience; (b) bridging applied and basic judgment/decision-making and capacity research; (c) focusing on new patient populations, such as individuals with developmental disabilities as they age; (d) strengthening assessment instruments and practices by gathering additional data on underrepresented groups (e.g., minorities, rural-dwelling individuals) or relating performance on assessment instruments to meaningful real-world functional performance criteria; (e) improving clinical education at the basic health care provider level; and (f) establishing effective communication about capacity issues across professional contexts. The series of American Bar Association/APA handbooks (2005, 2006, 2008) links civil capacity issues encountered by lawyers, judges, and psychologists. Other traditional medically oriented disciplines (e.g., primary care physicians, psychiatrists, surgeons, physician assistants, nurse practitioners), financial consultants (e.g., accountants, bankers, real estate agents) and allied health care specialists (including speech pathologists, pharmacists, and pastoral chaplains) also are more likely now than in prior generations to encounter greater numbers of older adult clients with diminished capacity and impaired decision making as a result of the demographic tsunami of the aging baby boomers. The greater number of professionals encountering older clients with impaired decision making further illustrates the need for more geropsychologists participating in collaborative care. This brings into play ethical issues with regard to human relations, particularly the importance of cooperating with other professionals (Standard 3.09).

The second area of ethical importance that geropsychologists must frequently consider in practice within civil and criminal forensic contexts is human relations. Geropsychologists must be mindful of unfair discrimination (Standard 3.01) with regard to assessment findings and psychometric normative comparisons when evaluating the civil or criminal capacity of an older adult self-identifying as a member of an underrepresented group. APA (2013) Guideline 2.08 (Appreciation of Individual and Group Differences) states,

> Forensic practitioners strive to understand how factors associated with age, gender, gender identity, race, ethnicity, culture, national origin, religion, sexual orientation, disability, language, socioeconomic status, or other relevant individual and cultural differences may affect and be related to the basis for people's contact and involvement with the legal system. Forensic practitioners do not engage in unfair discrimination based on such factors or on any basis proscribed by law. (p. 10)

Guideline 5 of the *Guidelines for Psychological Practice With Older Adults* (APA, 2014c) also identifies cohort and urban or rural residence among the issues that geropsychologists should consider when evaluating and treating older adults.

Particularly in criminal forensic contexts, the risk of unfair discrimination based on race/ethnicity is exacerbated by the disproportional number of inmates who self-identify as African American (Federal Bureau of Prisons, 2016b). These individuals may face greater discrimination and stigma in assessment and treatment settings that practice traditional care delivery models and deemphasize patient-centered care. APA (2013) Guideline 10.02 (Selection and Use of Assessment Procedures) states,

> Forensic practitioners use assessment instruments whose validity and reliability have been established for use with members of the population assessed. When such validity and reliability have not been established, forensic practitioners consider and describe the strengths and limitations of their findings. (p. 15)

Frequently, practicing geropsychologists develop "local norms" for comparison purposes to avoid the harm that can occur by making decisions based on culturally inappropriate comparison groups that differ significantly from the demographic characteristics of their own practice setting.

Moreover, Guideline 18 (APA, 2014c) and Standard 3.09 (Cooperation with Other Professionals) highlight the need for effective interprofessional communication and cooperation in working with older adults, particularly when services are delivered to or through organizations (Standard 3.11). Geropsychologists in general are particularly skilled in facilitating interdisciplinary services. Such facilitation must include becoming familiar with the roles of other professionals as well as educating other professionals about the potential role of psychologists, as evidence is accumulating that higher quality patient care outcomes occur when teams are interdisciplinary rather than multidisciplinary (Areán & Gum, 2013; O'Shea Carney et al., 2015). Provision of services in specialty settings such as jails or prisons necessitate knowledge of the setting's culture, institutional dynamics, and challenges in the provision of assessment and treatment of older adults, including ethical tensions between Principle A (Beneficence and Nonmaleficence) and Principle E (Respect for People's Rights and Dignity).

Notably, the United States incarcerates more individuals per capita than any other nation (Wilper et al., 2009), and according to the Federal Bureau of Prisons (2016a), 17.2% of the entire prison population in the United States is over the age of 50. This number is expected to increase rapidly over the next 5 years and is projected to reach 33% (Chettiar, Bunting, & Schotter, 2012). Carson (2014) summarized the demographic characteristics of federal and state prison inmates. By the end of 2013, 17% of all inmates (253,800) were ages 30 to 34, while an estimated 2% (31,900) were age 65 or older. Among males, White prisoners were generally older than Black or Hispanic prisoners; an estimated 17,300 inmates age 65 or older (54%) were White.

The third primary area of ethical importance that geropsychologists must frequently consider in forensic contexts involves privacy and confidentiality in assessment, treatment, and research. Maintaining privacy and confidentiality in forensic contexts may be challenging for geropsychologists because of requirements of the setting (e.g., presence of correctional officers, required sharing of information within the correctional setting) and the purposes for which the services are provided. The limits to privacy and confidentiality can be much different in forensic contexts than in common clinical contexts. In some forensic contexts it is expected and understood that the information or results obtained, regarding both assessment and treatment, will be conveyed to the retaining party or court and in some instances may become part of the public record. Geropsychologists have a responsibility to maintain confidentiality except as consented to by the examinee or retaining party or as permitted or required by law (Guideline 8, Privacy, Confidentiality, and Privilege; APA, 2013) and an obligation to inform examinees of the anticipated limits of confidentiality (Guideline 6, Informed Consent, Notification, and Assent; APA, 2013). Guideline 6.03, Communication With Forensic Examinees (APA, 2013) states,

> Forensic practitioners inform examinees about the nature and purpose of the examination. . . . Such information may include the purpose, nature, and anticipated use of the examination; who will have access to the information; associated limitations on privacy, confidentiality, and privilege including who is authorized to release or access the information contained in the forensic practitioner's records; the voluntary or involuntary nature of participation, including potential consequences of participation or nonparticipation, if known; and, if the cost of the service is the responsibility of the examinee, the anticipated cost. (pp. 12–13)

Geropsychologists understand that "the very conditions that precipitate psychological examination of individuals involved in legal proceedings can impair their functioning in a variety of important ways, including their ability to understand and consent to the evaluation process" (Guideline 6.03.03, Persons Lacking Capacity to Provide Informed Consent; APA, 2013) and take the necessary steps to obtain consent from the legally authorized person and obtain the examinee's assent to undergo the procedure.

For geropsychologists working in criminal forensic contexts, a potentially volatile topic involving Principle A (Beneficence and Nonmaleficence) versus Principle E (Respect for People's Rights and Dignity) is the issue of older inmates with diminished cognitive capacity on death row and the constitutionality of putting such individuals to death (Allen, Carden, & Salekin, 2015; Wood, Salekin, & Allen, 2014). Considerations of these two ethical principles in such context share variance; they are not conflicting. The very concepts of beneficence and nonmaleficence (Principle A) may be in question when considering what the most ethical outcome may be for such inmates: continued life on death row with cognitive incapacity or execution? In tandem, how does the ethical geropsychologist work to respect people's rights and dignity when the U.S. Supreme Court does not recognize cognitive incapacity among older inmates as a condition that precludes the death penalty? How could the rights and dignity of the cognitively impaired older inmate be maximized in such a context? The constitutionality of executions in relation to definitions of cruel and unusual punishment is, in effect, in question currently throughout the United States and not simply in reference to older prison inmates. Simply put, the potential implications of conducting a capacity assessment when the only outcome will be the State executing an older inmate regardless of his or her cognitive incapacity exponentially exacerbates ethical complexity and ethical considerations.

Given demographic trends, geropsychologists are likely to become more actively involved in the assessment and treatment of criminal forensic cases involving older offenders in the courts and in jail and prison contexts in the coming decades. For example, geropsychologists may be asked to assist counsel by evaluating whether the older adult has an understanding of the nature of the proceedings and the person's criminal responsibility (knowledge of right and wrong at the time the crime was committed). Given the average length of time inmates may spend on death row (17 years), initial questions of capacity in the context of trial may differ from an inmate's capacity to understand the death penalty and the purpose of retributive justice at or near the time of execution. Assessing an older inmate with diminished capacity for competence to be executed may directly pit Principle A (Beneficence and Nonmaleficence) against Principle E (Respect for People's Rights and Dignity), particularly in cases such as that of Scott Panetti. This case is discussed here as an example.

On December 3, 2014, the 5th U.S. Circuit Court of Appeals granted a stay of execution for Scott Panetti, an inmate diagnosed with paranoid schizophrenia and convicted of killing his in-laws in 1992 (Walker, 2014). Mr. Panetti was in the process of appealing a 2006 Circuit Court decision that found him, on the basis of the testimony of expert witnesses,

> to be aware that he would be executed, that he had committed the murders for which he was convicted and sentenced to death, and that the state's reason for executing him was that he had committed two murders. On this basis, the district court held that Mr. Panetti was competent to be executed. (Blanks & Pinals, 2007, p. 381)

Since that time, APA, the American Bar Association, the American Psychiatric Association, and the National Alliance on Mental Illness have passed resolutions recommending that individuals with severe mental illness be exempt from the death penalty ("Mental Illness and the Death Penalty," n.d.).

In such cases (e.g., Cecil Clayton, age 74, executed March 17, 2015), geropsychologists may be called upon to assess the cognitive capacity of older inmates to be ruled competent for execution or even to treat the inmate in an attempt to clear delusional belief systems, directly pitting Principle A (Beneficence and Nonmaleficence) against Principle E (Respect for People's Rights and Dignity; Blanks & Pinals, 2007; C. B. Fisher, 2012; Weinstock, Leong, & Silva, 2010). For example, geropsychologists have an ethical obligation to do no harm (nonmaleficence); however, if the older inmate is found, after a thorough assessment, to have the capacity to understand the issues, as was the case with Scott Panetti, then as a result of the geropsychologist's assessment findings the inmate can be put to death. For the inmate, then, the actions of the geropsychologist may be argued to have resulted in the greatest harm.

In contrast, from the perspective of benefit to society in general, as reflected in the ethical principle of general beneficence (Knapp & VandeCreek, 2006), the geropsychologist's assessment could be seen as providing evidence for the state to enact retributive justice, punishment proportionate to the crime as determined in a court of law. However, efforts to prioritize general versus specific beneficence are complex and controversial endeavors (see Chapter 3, this volume). Beauchamp and Childress (2013) maintained that "[t]he more widely we generalize obligations of beneficence, the less likely we will be to meet our primary responsibilities . . . the common morality recognizes significant limits to the demands of beneficence" (p. 205). Additionally, the potential value of distinguishing between similar and overlapping concepts, such as promotion of benefit (beneficence) versus the removal or prevention of harm, adds to the complexity of the issue (Beauchamp & Childress, 2013). Geropsychologists should strive to clarify these complex issues in terms of both their overall work in forensic contexts and their involvement with specific clients.

C. B. Fisher (2012) related death penalty litigation to the amendments to the APA (2010) Ethics Code Standard 1.02, Conflicts Between Ethics and Law, Regulations or Other Governing Legal Authority, that were enacted after the controversy regarding the role of psychologists practicing in military settings and potentially involved in or privy to the use of enhanced interrogation techniques. C. B. Fisher called for greater clarity in the Ethics Code regarding the role of forensic assessment in such cases. Geropsychologists are well served by overtly integrating their personal values into the ethical decision-making process, particularly in potentially controversial matters such as these, so that the influence of the values can be understood and their impact on ethical decision making taken into account.

To date, the U.S. Supreme Court has declined to hear any case that addresses the constitutionality of the death penalty for aged prisoners with diminished capacity, though such a case was brought to the Court in 2006 (i.e., Allen v. Ornoski), and the Court has established that certain individuals who lack the capacity to understand the nature of their crimes (e.g., those under the age of 18 at the time they committed the offense and those with intellectual disability [formerly referred to as *mental retardation*]) cannot be put to death because such action would constitute cruel and unusual punishment (Wood et al., 2014). Although the United States has declined to consider this issue, 14 countries across the world have excluded the elderly from a sentence of death (Center for International Human Rights at Northwestern University School of Law, 2011). Recent statistics show that more than 10% of the inmates (i.e., 315) on death row at the end of 2011 were age 60 and above (Wood et al., 2014).

The ethical issues for geropsychologists within this specific context are multifold and can be extremely complex (Blanks & Pinals, 2007; C. B. Fisher, 2012; Weinstock et al., 2010), but a basic assessment-related ethical issue concerns the geropsychologist's competence to assess cognitive capacity among older adults. This foundational assessment competency area is well-established in civil court and frequently encountered by geropsychologists in a variety of contexts. As stated in the *Specialty Guidelines for Forensic Psychology* (APA, 2013; Guideline 2.01, Scope of Competence):

> When determining one's competence to provide services in a particular matter, forensic practitioners may consider a variety of factors including the relative complexity and specialized nature of the service, relevant training and experience, the preparation and study they are able to devote to the matter, and the opportunity for consultation with a professional of established competence in the subject matter in question. (p. 9)

Geropsychologists need specialized training in those aspects of forensic practice in which they engage or are reasonably likely to engage at some point, such as decisional capacity assessments. Such forensic aspects of practice are commonly part of formal geropsychology training. For broader aspects of forensic psychology that are beyond the scope of competence for many geropsychologists, consultation with or referral to a psychology colleague who has more extensive training and experience in forensic matters is indicated.

Across civil and criminal forensic settings, geropsychologists must consider ethical issues arising from consultation. It is important (a) to establish and clarify with all parties who the client is, (b) to determine the nature and parameters of the services, and (c) to consider the need for modifications of standardized procedures and the possible impact that such divergence from standardized procedures could have on decisions made about the examinee. For example, the presence of a third party (e.g., correctional officer) in the examination room or behind one-way glass introduces a potential distraction that could affect test results and lead to erroneous conclusions (see McCaffrey, 2005, for a review). Additionally, examinees who are required to wear handcuffs may have their performance on visuospatial and other motor tasks adversely affected or negated, requiring the geropsychologist to temper conclusions accordingly.

> Assessment in forensic contexts differs from assessment in therapeutic contexts in important ways that forensic practitioners strive to take into account when conducting forensic examinations. Forensic practitioners seek to consider the strengths and limitations of employing traditional assessment procedures in forensic examinations. . . . Forensic practitioners consider and seek to make known that forensic examination results can be affected by factors unique to, or differentially present in, forensic contexts including response style, voluntariness of participation, and situational stress associated with involvement in forensic or legal matters. (APA, 2013; Guideline 10.02, p. 15)

Vignette

A geropsychologist is asked to complete a forensic evaluation of a 62-year-old inmate on death row in a state prison to provide information about his cognitive capacity to understand his sentence, which will be used to determine his competency for execution. The inmate was sentenced to death for the murder of an elderly couple for whom he worked in 1994, and he has been on death row since that time, spending up to 23 hours a day alone in his cell. At the time of his sentencing, the inmate showed no remorse for his crime, and the children and grandchildren of his victims vowed to be present, if possible, at the time of his execution. In the past 3 years, the inmate has exhibited increasing confusion and decline in functional abilities, including bathing, dressing, and grooming. The results of the clinical interview and assessment reveal that he has moderate dementia and that he is variably aware of his sentence, although he does remember his actions in murdering the elderly couple and reports feelings of remorse for his "greedy, mean ways" as a younger man. The geropsychologist is ambivalent about arriving at a conclusion that could result in the inmate's execution and considers whether emphasizing the inmate's periods of lack of awareness of his sentence might better serve the interests of justice.

Ethical Issues, Tensions, and Resources

Convicted criminals sentenced to death must be competent for execution before they can be executed (Ford v. Wainwright, 1986). Geropsychologists are sometimes asked by the courts to assist in determinations of competency for execution. Performing such evaluations raises ethical and moral concerns among some practitioners. This geropsychologist experiences tension between Principle A (Beneficence and Nonmaleficence) and Principle E

(Respect for People's Rights and Dignity). The desire to want to be helpful to both the inmate and the legal system elicits the geropsychologist's personal feelings and values. She understands that her conclusions could lead to the inmate's death and wonders how this situation could possibly be consistent with her primary ethical responsibility to do no harm. She wonders whether professional competence to perform this type of evaluation (Standard 2.01) is adequate or whether a certain moral stance might also be required as part of, or in addition to, professional competence in this setting. When considering whether she might be able to rely on the Ethics Code to justify to herself her hesitancy to offer an opinion that could result in the inmate being executed in accordance with his sentence, she finds the following statement from Standard 1.02 (Conflicts Between Ethics and Law, Regulations or Other Governing Legal Authority) to be particularly interesting: "Under no circumstances may this standard be used to justify or defend violating human rights." However, she then wonders whose rights would be applicable in her situations, those of the inmate or those of the murdered persons and their families.

Geropsychologists strive to remain open, aware, and engaged in ongoing self-assessment of the boundaries of their competence (Standard 2.01). Additionally, Guideline 2 of the *Guidelines for Psychological Practice With Older Adults* (APA, 2014c) states that geropsychologists recognize how their own attitudes and beliefs about aging may be relevant to assessment and treatment. The geropsychologist understands that the court rather than the inmate is her client (Standard 3.07, Third Party Request for Services). Although the court simply wants to establish the inmate's cognitive capacity to understand the nature of his sentence and has no preference regarding whether the inmate has capacity, the geropsychologist nevertheless is aware that all stakeholders, except the inmate, want the execution to occur. Indeed, the functional abilities that she believes are most important in determinations of competency for execution may not be the same as those the judge is likely to consider most informative (Ackerson, Brodsky, & Zapf, 2005; Demakis, 2012). For example, judges tend to give more weight to legal issues, such as the inmate's knowledge of the crime that he was convicted of and sentenced for, than to clinical issues such as the severity of a mental defect, although the clinical issues are also considered important (Ackerson et al., 2005). The geropsychologist's knowledge of dementia and interpretation of test results may put her in a bind between what she believes the court and others want and her knowledge that her evaluation results have direct implications for the life of a man who faces the death penalty for a 21-year-old crime. She has an ethical responsibility (Principle D, Justice) to take reasonable precautions to ensure that her personal biases do not lead to or condone unjust practices; if she cannot do that, she should excuse herself from the case and likely from work in this type of setting. Bush, Connell, and Denney (2006) argued that "it is the forensic psychologist's responsibility to thoroughly and adequately perform his or her duties; if the resultant outcome favors the 'unjust,' we believe that the psychologist must forgo a sense of personal responsibility for that injustice" (p. 18).

Former APA president Donald Bersoff, PhD, in a 2013 President's Column, called for APA to take a stand against the death penalty. He argued that while criminals should be held accountable for their actions, retributive punishment is essentially sanctioned vengeance and therefore should not be tolerated in a civilized society. He concluded, "the death penalty is indefensible from a scientific perspective, and arguing for its abolition is the moral and ethical thing to do" (Bersoff, 2013, p. 5). Celia B. Fisher, chair of the 2002 revision of the Ethics Code, stated that given the flaws inherent in psychological evaluations (e.g., cultural bias, dealing in probabilities), "psychologists' participation in capital cases is ethically troubling" and that "psychologists' contribution to legal decisions concerning competency and predictions of future violence hearings places the defendant at the mercy of an imperfect and unjust system," which at times violates the basic human rights to life and liberty by killing innocent persons (C. B. Fisher, 2013). In the context of negotiating the ethical and moral conflicts experienced when performing competency for execution examinations, Neal (2010) suggested that practitioners, in the context of "capacity for execution" assessments, remain mindful that their opinions are just that—opinions—rather than legal dispositions.

The geropsychologist must be clear with the inmate about her role, the intended recipients of the assessment information, and the implications of the results of this assessment (Standard 3.11, Psychological Services Delivered to or Through Organizations). Although the geropsychologist may strive to describe the situation as clearly as possible, it may be that the inmate's current cognitive deficits diminish his ability to fully understand the nature of the assessment and its possible consequences.

Preferred Course of Action

The geropsychologist should carefully consider whether her personal values allow her the objectivity needed to perform this type of evaluation in this setting. If so, she should perform an appropriate evaluation and in her conclusions rely as heavily as possible on the objective assessment results. Consultation with trusted peers who are experts in death penalty assessment would enhance the geropsychologist's ability to perform competently and objectively in her retained role. If she determines that such objectivity is not possible given her personal values, she should decline the case and seek work in settings that are more in keeping with her values and her commitment to doing no harm.

HOSPICE AND PALLIATIVE CARE

Overview

All end-of-life decisions have complex psychosocial components that affect the quality of living and dying, and psychologists play a meaningful role in hospice, palliative care, and other settings in which end-of-life needs are addressed. The World Health Organization (1996) defined *hospice and palliative care* as meeting the physical, psychosocial, and spiritual needs of patients with life-limiting and advanced chronic illness and their families through an interprofessional approach that improves comfort and quality of life (Campbell & Amin, 2012). The focus of palliative care is on the prevention and relief of suffering through early identification and treatment of physical, psychosocial, and spiritual problems. Discussions regarding goals of care and the potential of death often occur very late in the disease process or not at all (Bailey et al., 2012; Connors et al., 1995; Guo et al., 2010). Notably, medical providers are not particularly accurate with prognostication regarding the disease trajectory of chronic illness, sometimes incorrectly estimating an individual's time left to live by a factor of up to five (Chow et al., 2001; Christakis & Lamont, 2000; Stiel et al., 2010).

With regard to the Death With Dignity movement, five states have now legislated Death With Dignity acts (Oregon in 1997, Washington in 2008, Vermont in 2013, New Jersey in 2014, and California in 2015), and one state (Montana) supports physician-assisted death through common law ("Death With Dignity Around the US," 2016). Death With Dignity acts allow competent and terminally ill adult residents of that state to voluntarily request and receive a prescription medication to hasten their death. Additional states are considering such legislation. Perhaps in no other aspect of practice do ethical considerations involve more personal values for geropsychologists than in working with older adults approaching the end of life. The ethical considerations commonly include respect for patient autonomy, conflicts between ethics and law, professional competence, and human relations.

Particularly in states that do not currently have Death With Dignity acts, geropsychologists working with older adults and their families near the end of life may encounter conflicts between ethics and law (Standard 1.02, Conflicts Between Ethics and Law, Regulations, or Other Governing Legal Authority). In these situations, the geropsychologist must balance Principle A (Beneficence and Nonmaleficence) with Principle E (Respect for People's Rights and Dignity) and consider the ramifications of acting in accordance with mandatory reporting laws if confronted with a coherent plan by the terminally ill client to end his or her own life. Preferably, the geropsychologist would be able to work with the patient and family to consider hospice as an alternative treatment option.

These advance planning discussions have direct benefit for the patient and family, and the execution of advance directives and engagement in advance care planning prior to a health crisis is recommended. Reimbursement for physicians or other health care providers such as geropsychologists to counsel older individuals about their medical care rights, however, was excluded from the 2010 Patient Protection and Affordable Care Act, Medicare wellness visits, and Centers for Medicare and Medicaid Services practice guidelines due to public concern regarding "death panels" (Tinetti, 2012).

Within the context of palliative care and hospice settings, treatment planning conversations are ongoing and will become more frequent within primary care with the aging of the baby boomer cohort. First and foremost, geropsychologists ensure that they provide competent services to their older clients by seeking consultation or referring to colleagues when issues arise outside of their practice area (Standard 2.01, Boundaries of Competence). Because training programs do not routinely require exposure to and competent performance in assessment and intervention with individuals near the end of life, geropsychologists may face ethical challenges with regard to their competence to practice in this domain (Standards 2.01 and 2.04). According to the *Guidelines for Psychological Practice With Older Adults* (APA, 2014c), geropsychologists strive to increase their knowledge, understanding, and skills in new practice areas throughout their careers (Guideline 21). When the geropsychologist determines that he or she lacks the competence to provide ethical care to individuals near the end of life, referral is appropriate (Standard 2.01b). If the geropsychologist works in a setting in which such a referral is not possible, he or she "with closely related prior training or experience may provide such services in order to ensure that services are not denied if they make a reasonable effort to obtain the competence required by using relevant research, training, consultation, or study" (Standard 2.01d).

Geropsychologists working with older individuals near the end of life should also consider the ethical standards involving human relations (Standards 3.01, 3.04, and 3.09). Geropsychologists strive to avoid harm (Standard 3.04) and unfair discrimination (Standard 3.01) through practice that is culturally competent and applicable to a variety of underrepresented groups. Geropsychologists working in palliative care and hospice settings of necessity must work with interdisciplinary teams (Standard 3.09, Cooperation With Other Professionals). Particularly when working in an area rife with divergent personal values such as end-of-life care, differing ethical priorities across disciplines and lack of understanding of the roles of specific team members may result in ineffective communication and conflict (Engel & Prentice, 2013; Mitchell, Parker, Giles, & Boyle, 2014). Mitchell et al. (2014), however, found that dysfunctional interdisciplinary team functioning was minimized within the context of transformational leadership, reinforcement of shared values and goals, and the development of a shared group identity. Transformational leadership motivates group members by increasing their awareness of the importance of designated goals and aligning their personal values with the team's collective vision (Bass, 1985). Traditionally, hospice and palliative care interdisciplinary team meetings strive to promote shared values and goals (e.g., assisting the individual to die with dignity). Unfortunately, psychology still is underrepresented in palliative care and hospice settings, which frequently involve only medicine, nursing, social work, and clergy (Haley, Larson, Kasl-Godley, Neimeyer, & Kwilosz, 2003). Training opportunities at the predoctoral and particularly the internship and postdoctoral levels, however, are increasing, enabling geropsychologists to bring to bear their skills in interdisciplinary care and communication to palliative and hospice settings (Allen, Noh, Beck, & Smith, 2016).

Vignette

A 69-year-old male patient and his 74-year-old female partner of 45 years reside in a small city in Texas. The patient was diagnosed with acute leukemia just over 1 year ago and has been seeing a geropsychologist since that time to deal with issues of anticipatory grief and advance care planning. As expected, the patient's physical condition has rapidly deteriorated, and he is now receiving hospice care from one of only two hospice agencies serving his geographic region. His partner is his primary caregiver. His only living relative is a sister who refused contact with him after he came out a "trans man" (female-to-male transgendered individual) when he was 28 years old.

Throughout his adult lifetime, the patient has been consistent with his hormone replacement therapy and presentation as a masculine gender. The patient related early in therapy with the geropsychologist that though his relationship with his partner is excellent, his life as a trans man in Texas has been peppered with discrimination and a lack of acceptance and understanding in some work and social settings (e.g., church). Now, nearing the end of his life and engaging in reminiscence therapy with the geropsychologist, he thinks that forgiving those who discriminated against him would allow him to release some persisting anger and face his final days more peacefully. However, such efforts are a struggle.

During an in-home session, the patient tells the geropsychologist that he is becoming increasingly frustrated with the hospice nurse who visits once weekly to check on his pain levels and the effectiveness of the analgesic medication. He reports to the geropsychologist that other than his primary care physician, he and his partner have encountered discrimination by health care providers throughout their relationship. He stated, "At first they seem warm, genuinely concerned, and willing to discuss treatment plans with us, but once they discover my trans identity they become distant and reserved." His partner, having entered the room several minutes earlier, tells the geropsychologist that she typically receives minimal eye contact and gets terse answers to her questions about how to provide the best comfort care for the patient at home or whether there is a local inpatient hospice unit available should the patient's needs increase. Both the patient and his partner relate that they feel that the nursing aides who come into the home to help the patient shower and dress often treat him with disrespect and cast looks of disgust toward what they view as incongruities between his physical body and gender presentation. The patient and his partner ask the geropsychologist if he can intervene with the hospice staff or administration to attempt to improve the quality of care provided to the patient. The geropsychologist is in independent practice but has received and provided referrals to this hospice organization for the past 3 years. He wants to help but does not want to start problems with staff that could have a lasting effect on his relationships with them or the hospice organization, or that could bring retaliatory mistreatment to the patient.

Ethical Issues, Tensions, and Resources

The geropsychologist must balance his desire to remedy the apparent unfair discrimination (beneficence) and his desire to cooperate with other professionals (Standard 3.09, Cooperation With Other Professionals) employed by this hospice, one of only two serving clients in this small city in Texas, with his concerns about retaliatory mistreatment of the patient's partner and possibly harming his relationships with other hospice workers. It may be that the geropsychologist's own personal attitude toward gender identity and expression is relatively open and in line with Principles E (Respect for People's Rights and Dignity) and D (Justice). This personal and professional stance may motivate the geropsychologist to consider requesting a meeting with the executive director of this hospice to discuss the issues and offer to provide in-service training for hospice staff on transgender identities. However, the geropsychologist is also aware that limited resources in this small Texas city may make it difficult to find better alternative treatment if the consultation goes poorly. Moreover, the referrals the geropsychologist has received from this hospice have been increasing in the past 3 years.

Particular ethical tensions for the geropsychologist include the commitment to helping the patient and his partner while avoiding bringing or causing harm to them (Standard 3.04, Avoiding Harm), as well as attempting to cooperate with other professionals (Standard 3.09, Cooperation With Other Professionals) in addressing issues of perceived unfair discrimination without jeopardizing currently productive working relationships. It could be that any action on the geropsychologist's part could place at risk both the patient's ability to receive in-home hospice care in this small city and the geropsychologist's own business by potentially reducing referrals from this organization.

APA has developed several sets of guidelines to encourage psychologists to monitor and reduce or eliminate the impact of personal bias on professional activities, including the Ethics Code, *Guidelines for Psychotherapy With Lesbian, Gay and Bisexual Clients* (APA, 2012b), and *Guidelines for Psychological Practice With Older Adults* (APA, 2014c). Additionally, general resources that are not specific to the discipline of geropsychology are available through the website of the National Hospice and Palliative Care Organization (http://www.nhpco.org/). Although these resources provide a wealth of information, no specific guidelines for dealing specifically with potential discrimination against trans-identified individuals currently exist within APA.

Preferred Course of Action

The geropsychologist should work closely with the patient and his partner while the couple is able to engage in informed and shared decision making, with the goal of completing an advance directive and clarifying their desired plan for the patient's end-of-life health care. Additionally, the geropsychologist should attempt to meet with the leadership and staff of this local hospice program to offer training in working with trans-identified individuals near the end of life. Participating in such an interprofessional meeting may enhance communication between the geropsychologist and hospice staff as well as provide needed continuing education for the hospice staff on a topic of increasing importance. Such a meeting would also illustrate the geropsychologist's commitment to cooperating with other professionals (Standard 3.09). The risk of harming the relationship between the hospice program and the geropsychologist is worth the geropsychologist's need to advocate for the patient. Although more referrals from this hospice program may indeed serve a salutary public service in this community by yielding more psychological care to hospice patients, the proximal beneficent needs of this identified patient overrides such distal possibilities. Open communication from a position of mutual respect and investment in patient care may well meet the needs of all parties.

As a matter of practice in working with individuals and their families near the end of life, the geropsychologist should also engage in ongoing self-assessment of personal values and biases. Perhaps in no other practice setting than in situations of life and death is a geropsychologist's commitment to openness, awareness, and involvement in the process of interpersonal engagement and professional competence so important.

CONCLUSION

Geropsychologists provide wide-ranging services in diverse practice settings. Although general ethical principles and many specific ethical standards are relevant across settings, the emphases placed on various ethical issues and challenges vary according to the setting and context in which services are provided, and some ethical issues are setting specific. This chapter presented a sample of practice settings and contexts in which geropsychologists practice and described common ethical issues and challenges associated with those contexts. The following contexts were covered: primary care, hospital units, home-based care, long-term care, forensic contexts, and hospice and palliative care. Geropsychologists must understand the ethical issues that pertain to their practice settings and the challenges that are likely to be encountered in those settings. The risk of ethical pitfalls increases when changing from one setting or context to another. It is particularly important during such changes to strive to understand the ethical issues and challenges that are likely to be encountered in the new setting.

9

ADVOCACY IN GEROPSYCHOLOGY: PROMOTING SERVICES AND PROTECTING RIGHTS

What one does is what counts and not what one had the intention of doing.
—Pablo Picasso

Advocacy in geropsychology is not a single activity, is not performed on behalf of a single person or group, and is not performed in a single type of setting. There are wide-ranging advocacy opportunities for geropsychologists: on behalf of others, organizations, institutions, and even the practice of geropsychology. Common specific types of advocacy for geropsychologists, which are covered in this chapter, include (a) advocacy for the older clients being served, (b) advocacy for older adults and their families, (c) advocacy for improved geriatric business practices and insurance reimbursement policies, and (d) advocacy for changes in institutional procedures for the betterment of aged residents. For each type of advocacy, ethical principles that guide a geropsychologist's advocacy work are presented. A case vignette highlights the ethical principles encountered at the intersection of geropsychological clinical activities and advocacy.

Despite substantial advocacy work at the national and state psychological association levels addressing geriatric mental health, and the pervasive

http://dx.doi.org/10.1037/0000010-010
Ethical Practice in Geropsychology, by S. S. Bush, R. S. Allen, and V. A. Molinari

view that influencing public policy can improve the lives of older adults (Hinrichsen, Kietzman, et al., 2010), surprisingly little has been written about how to advocate effectively and which ethical principles should inform these activities. Just as with administration and the business aspects of psychology, it seems that advocacy is something that is expected to bloom spontaneously upon licensure, with little training necessary for effective practice other than perhaps the observation and modeling of esteemed senior colleagues in action. One bright spot is the "Standards for Psychological Services in Long-Term Care Facilities" (Lichtenberg et al., 1998):

> Psychologists advocate for the appropriate use of mental health services to reduce excess disability and improve quality of life. . . . When mental health services are being used inappropriately, psychologists strive to educate other care providers to improve the delivery of care in order to be consistent with a biopsychosocial approach to the assessment and treatment of older adults. (p. 126)

The American Psychological Association (APA; 2014e) states that education and training in psychology uniquely positions psychologists to contribute to the development of federal policies and programs.

Unfortunately, in other seminal writings in geropsychology, advocacy is barely mentioned or is just given short shrift. In the widely cited paper on the Pikes Peak model of training, Knight et al. (2009) merely suggested that geropsychologists "apply scientific knowledge to geropsychology practice and policy advocacy" (p. 213). In the application for APA specialty status, under the section on Consumer Protection, it is simply noted that geropsychologists "advocate for better social conditions, health care, and other programs and care systems for older adults" (p. 14). Furthermore, the American Board of Professional Psychology in geropsychology does not test for competence in advocacy. Indeed, although some sections of the *Ethical Principles of Psychologists and Code of Conduct* (hereinafter, Ethics Code; APA, 2010) are relevant, there are no specific APA ethical principles or standards that address advocacy per se. Given the paucity of writings on advocacy for geropsychology and geriatric mental health, we thought it useful to introduce ethical issues that reflect tensions involved in balancing competing principles.

SPECIFIC TYPES OF ADVOCACY ACTIVITIES

Advocacy for the Older Clients One Serves

Advocacy for the older adult clients that geropsychologists serve can take many forms. At the most basic level, this type of advocacy entails a geropsychologist working with a client and recognizing that the system in which the service is provided is failing to meet the client's needs. In outpatient geriatric mental health settings, the person may be "falling through the cracks of the system" and unable to access the proper transportation, health care, food, housing, and other needs. In such situations, the geropsychologist may begin to functionally operate as a geriatric care manager trying to access or coordinate needed services. Although interdisciplinary teamwork and integrated care is an important part of a geropsychologist's training and is always to be fostered (Areán & Gum, 2013; Zeiss & Steffen, 1996), conflicts and turf wars between disciplines may arise when there is not a designated team and the client is not receiving necessary services. At such times, the geropsychologist may be crossing paths or even stepping on the toes of professionals from other disciplines who may not be fulfilling their duties with the client. More likely, the fractionated health care system is to blame, and the geropsychologist must temporarily take on neglected roles and do a warm hand-off to the health care professional who finally understands and accepts the responsibility to carry on these tasks. In these situations, geropsychologists are guided by a section of Principle A (Beneficence and Nonmaleficence):

> Psychologists consult with, refer to, or cooperate with other professionals and institutions to the extent needed to serve the best interests of those with whom they work. They are concerned about the ethical compliance of their colleagues' scientific and professional conduct.

Across the geriatric setting spectrum, suspicions of elder abuse frequently trigger client advocacy considerations. As is well-known, elder abuse frequently occurs within a "shared living situation" (Lachs & Pillemer, 2004, p. 1265), and older persons often have attachments to the abuser and fear that if the abuse is reported they will be removed from their homes or treated more harshly by the abuser. In such situations, geropsychological decision making must be dictated by state laws and reporting requirements, but the general emphasis of Principle A (Beneficence and Nonmaleficence) comes into play in those gray areas whereby specific clinical courses of action are not clear-cut, and the geropsychologist must gauge the consequences of disruptions in the therapeutic relationship and the dearth of viable alternate housing arrangements.

Geropsychologists frequently find themselves working in institutional settings where they feel it incumbent on them to advocate for their client's individual needs. For example, a nursing home resident may complain that the food is unsavory, the aides are loud at night, or the bathing time is inconvenient. Geropsychologists must then balance the needs of the resident with the practicalities of communal living and often scarce nursing home resources. Determining what is best for the specific resident, what most of the other residents desire, and what best suits the needs of the institution can be tricky. But once again psychologists are guided by Principle A (Beneficence and

Nonmaleficence): "When conflicts occur among psychologists' obligations or concerns, they attempt to resolve these conflicts in a responsible fashion that avoids or minimizes harm."

Finally, discriminatory policies may affect the well-being of older clients, and the multiculturally competent geropsychologist must be aware of how to address diversity issues (Hinrichsen, 2006) and how to advocate on the local level for the specific patient. APA (2004) includes age as a diversity factor, and many older adults have dual or triple minority status affiliations (e.g., an older Latina woman who is also a lesbian). In addition to the general adaptations that should commonly be made on behalf of older adults in assessment (Edelstein et al., 2008) or treatment (Knight, 2004), geropsychologists should incorporate sociocultural considerations in their clinical formulations (Hinrichsen, 2006). Geropsychologists working with diverse clients are guided by APA's *Guidelines on Multicultural Education, Training, Research, Practice, and Organizational Change for Psychologists* (2003), *Guidelines for Psychological Practice With Older Adults* (APA, 2004), and Principle E (Respects for People's Rights and Dignity). The latter states,

> Psychologists are aware of and respect cultural, individual and role differences, including those based on age, gender, gender identity, race, ethnicity, culture, national origin, religion, sexual orientation, disability, language and socioeconomic status and consider these factors when working with members of such groups.

General Advocacy for the Mental Health of Older Adults and Their Families

Many geropsychologists write letters to their congressional representatives, others participate in White House Conference on Aging regional meetings, and some even provide testimony to Congress on issues involving funding for the National Institute on Aging and the National Institute of Mental Health or involving support for those with Alzheimer's disease and their caregivers. In general, this is the type of advocacy with which the public and most psychologists are familiar. Much of this advocacy is done in conjunction with state psychological associations, and collaboration with local stakeholders appears essential for successful outcomes (Hinrichsen, Kietzman, et al., 2010; see also APA, 2014d). At these times, psychologists serve as representatives of their profession and should be guided by their ethos as both practitioners and scientists. In adhering to Principle B (Fidelity and Responsibility) guidance that psychologists are "aware of their professional and scientific responsibilities to society and to the specific communities in which they work," geropsychologists must be careful to convey their often emotion-laden messages in an effective manner without compromising their scientific integrity.

Geropsychologists often conduct public advocacy for older adults and their family members by writing columns or editorials on age-related concerns, being interviewed about geriatric issues, or giving talks on the mental health of older adults. By virtue of their education and training, geropsychologists are in a good position to advocate for more funding for aging services, but care is needed not to highlight one-sidedly the negatives and frailties of aging without also discussing the benefits, such as wisdom, that may accrue with the aging process. Such public advocacy is definitely needed, but in keeping with Principle C (Integrity), geropsychologists must "promote accuracy, honesty, and truthfulness."

To stir up grassroots advocacy, geropsychologists may educate the general public regarding myths about aging; normal aging stressors; late life transitions; and how to cope with retirement, caregiving, physical impairment, and bereavement by engaging in meaningful activities and developing and maintaining social relationships. These didactic activities may be viewed as preventative strategies that might alert older adults and family members about developmental challenges to stave off adjustment disorders and even florid mental health symptoms by facilitating aging transitions in psychologically healthy age-appropriate and resilient ways. These professional activities can serve the dual purpose of providing the aging public and its members' caregivers with resources, while the geropsychologist may garner referrals in the community by being identified as an expert in this area. Community service presentations also may help fulfill an aspect of Principle D (Justice), which notes that "fairness and justice entitle all persons to access to and benefit from the contributions of psychology and to equal quality in the processes."

One final topic within this category that must be considered is advocacy for the informal caregivers of those with dementia. As is well-known, family caregivers spend inordinate amounts of time, energy, and finances to assist their loved ones when cognitive processes are declining. If they were not to do so, the burden would fall to society through increased government expenditures as a result of greater Medicaid costs and more emergency room visits to assist this vulnerable population. Family caregivers do this out of a sense of loyalty to their loved ones, but the burdens put upon them can have multilevel consequences: emotional (caregivers are more likely to be depressed), social (caregivers tend to be unable to sustain friendships), vocational (caregivers often can only take part-time work), and financial (dementia is a very expensive disease; APA, 2014a). When the person with dementia dies, spousal or adult child caregivers may not be able to recoup their cost outlays and may be in more precarious financial conditions regarding their retirement income because of lower Social Security benefits and missed job promotions. This situation is especially salient in the lives of female caregivers, who make up the majority of caregivers and frequently earn less than their male counterparts. Advocacy for government programs to provide assistance to caregivers supports humane social policy and is in keeping with Principle D (Justice).

Advocacy for Training in Geriatric Mental Health

One area of particular advocacy concern is the tremendous need for increased training in geriatric mental health. It has been heartening that the Hartford Foundation has sponsored geriatric social work, nursing, and medical training over the years. However, it is surprising that with the aging demographic demand, approximately half of the geriatric residency medicine and geriatric psychiatry slots are going unfilled (Boulton, 2014; Institute of Medicine, 2012). Indeed, despite the need for high-quality mentoring in geropsychology (Zimmerman, Fiske, & Scogin, 2011) and an evidence-based link between the availability of specialty programs in geropsychology and later engagement in geropsychology-related professional activities across four countries (Woodhead et al., 2013), the number of graduate programs in the United States with major areas of study in geropsychology has not increased over the years.

This trend is particularly troubling given the demographic need for a trained geropsychology workforce that has gone unmet despite years of documentation (Hoge, Karel, Zeiss, Alegria, & Moye, 2015; Institute of Medicine, 2012; Qualls, Segal, Norman, Niederehe, & Gallagher-Thompson, 2002). Furthermore, funds specifically earmarked for geropsychology training within the Graduate Psychology Education program were terminated some years ago. APA has pushed national advocacy, especially for the latter initiative; conducted training in how to meet with members of Congress; and scheduled appointments with psychologists' representatives to put practice into action. The need for such advocacy is tempered by the time-consuming demands of conducting it (and perhaps also the financial requisites of donating to key congressional champions), but in keeping with Principle B (Fidelity and Responsibility): "Psychologists strive to contribute a portion of their professional time for little or no compensation or personal advantage."

Advocacy for Improved Business Practice and Insurance Reimbursement Policies

Advocacy for improved business practices is not unique to geropsychologists but remains strikingly important for the survival of geropsychology as a profession. At a variety of levels, geropsychologists have lobbied to increase reimbursement for Medicare to better serve older adults in nursing home settings. Perhaps the highest-profile successful advocacy effort has been in reducing the amount of copayment that insurance companies charge for mental health services to comparable 20% levels for those with "medical" problems. Two geropsychology leaders in particular, Norris (2008) and Hartman-Stein (Hartman-Stein & Ergun, 1998; Hartman-Stein & Georgoulakis, 2008), using different venues, have been staunch geropsychology advocates for psychologists' involvement in the political arena so that reimbursement rates are commensurate with doctorate-level education. For example, Dr. Norris has worked with the APA's Committee on Aging and the varied geropsychology organization e-mail lists to inform members how to conduct ethically sound business practices. Additionally, Dr. Hartman-Stein, writing a regular column for the *National Psychologist*, has used this independent practice forum to promote proper use of billing codes and documentation.

Years ago, geropsychology was dealt a setback when the Office of the Inspector General issued a blistering report decrying psychologists who conducted unnecessary extensive testing and group therapy with residents who were incapable of benefitting from such services (Norris, 2008, p. 4). Such behaviors dramatically conflict with aspects of Principle B: Fidelity and Responsibility and Principle C: Integrity which state, respectively, that psychologists "uphold professional standards of conduct" and "do not steal, cheat or engage in fraud, subterfuge or intentional misrepresentation of fact." It is unclear whether those psychologists involved in such activities were indeed participating in intentional fraud, but obviously they were not adhering to guidelines related to the boundaries of their competence especially with regard to Principle D (Justice), which states: "Psychologists exercise reasonable judgment and take precautions to ensure that their potential biases, the boundaries of their competence and the limitations of their expertise do not lead to or condone unjust practices." Unfortunately, when a small minority of psychologists engage in such behavior, the effects can be widespread.

Advocacy for Changes in Long-Term Care Institutional Policy

Although geropsychologists working in nursing homes have been in the forefront of developing humanistic person-centered assessment strategies (Mast, 2011), implementing evidence-based interventions for the treatment of behavioral problems of residents (Burgio & Kowalkowski, 2011; Camp & Lee, 2011; Cohen-Mansfield, Marx, Dakheel-Ali, & Thein, 2015), and conducting program evaluations of treatment strategies on a national level (Karlin, Visnic, Shealy McGee, & Teri, 2014), dissemination of these programs has lagged far behind the science. Indeed, the recent Centers for Medicare and Medicaid Services (CMS) initiative to reduce antipsychotic medication use by 15% for residents with dementia seemed tailor-made for psychologists to take center stage. However, this was not the case; CMS officials were more receptive to behaviorally based nonpsychopharmacological approaches only after repeated contacts with psychologists during which they explained what they have to offer. CMS is not to be blamed; geropsychologists must do a better job of "selling psychology" and disseminating our knowledge, so that the benefits of geropsychology can become readily apparent. Indeed, there are far more physicians, nurses, social workers, and other professionals working in long-term care settings than there are geropsychologists, and we must be more effective in communicating what we have to offer.

The CMS initiative was the culmination of more than 25 years of lobbying by long-term care advocates to induce nursing homes to conform to the spirit of the Omnibus Budget Reconciliation Act (1987). This legislation was an attempt to humanize the nursing home environment by (a) triaging inappropriate admissions to nursing homes into the community (e.g., those with serious mental illness and those with developmental disabilities), (b) eliminating the use of restraints (both physical and chemical), and (c) reducing the use of antipsychotic medications and promoting nonpsychopharmacological approaches as a first-line strategy in managing behavior problems. Geropsychologists trained in long-term care have the tools necessary to make a difference, but they must function within their local nursing home settings to assure that these techniques are used correctly. They must deftly negotiate a balance between what is in the best interests of the residents and the finite resources within which nursing homes have to operate. Given the high turnover rate for nursing home staff, training in behavioral principles and the maintenance of this training are ongoing expenses that some nursing homes may be loath to expend. However, even when a decision is made to work within a system that is not optimal, the geropsychologist should be guided by Principle A (Beneficence and Nonmaleficence), which states in part: "Because psychologists' scientific and professional judgments and actions may affect the lives of others, they are alert to and guard against personal, financial, social, organizational or political factors that might lead to misuse of their influence." Additionally, Principle B (Fidelity and Responsibility) is relevant: psychologists "uphold professional standards of conduct, clarify their professional roles and obligations, accept appropriate responsibility for their behavior and seek to manage conflicts of interest that could lead to exploitation or harm."

Another area of long-term care where psychologists have been at the scientific forefront is in the planning of the institutional milieu. Lawton (1983) reconceptualized an individual's disabilities as flaws in environmental planning, championing the need for a match between the person and the milieu of their residence. Rather than emphasizing the limitations of nursing home residents, this conceptual flip put the onus on architects and administrative personnel to fashion elder settings that satisfy the needs of frail residents with physical and cognitive impairments. A behavior "problem" is thereby not localized within the resident as an attribute of the disease but is viewed as an error of organizational design that needs mending at a higher level. Indeed, the "culture change" movement has made us aware that shifting nurse assignments, rigid scheduling of feeding and toileting, no pets, overly sanitized surroundings, and a medicalized hierarchical structure of care may be efficient but lack the features promoting quality of life and the flourishing of residents living in true homelike environments. A section of Principle E (Respect for People's Rights and Dignity) is particularly operative regarding the "humanizing" of long-term care: "Psychologists are aware that special safeguards may be necessary to protect the rights and welfare of persons or communities whose vulnerabilities impair autonomous decision making."

On a related note, frail older adults who live in nursing homes are often terminally ill, which bespeaks the need for advocacy for palliative care (Kasl-Godley, King, & Quill, 2014) and hospice in nursing home settings whereby residents are given truly informed choices regarding the status of their medical conditions and the options that are available to achieve the kind of "good death" that they (and their families) so desire. Geropsychologists trained in thanatological (study of death) issues may play a big role in helping dying residents choose how they want to lead the last days of their lives, assessing their tolerance for pain, honoring their religious or spiritual beliefs, and facilitating anticipatory grief work for family members in the dying process. Finally, changes in institutional policy regarding the humane, person-centered treatment of older adults in correctional facilities and state psychiatric hospitals should be noted as proper domains for advocacy. In these situations, Principle E (Respect for People's Rights and Dignity) directs geropsychologists to

> respect the dignity and worth of all people, and the rights of individuals to privacy, confidentiality, and self-determination. Psychologists are aware that special safeguards may be necessary to protect the rights and welfare of persons or communities whose vulnerabilities impair autonomous decision making.

VIGNETTE

A geropsychologist provides outpatient and in-home services to older adults living in a continuing care retirement community which is located just a few miles away from his office. An 84-year-old White, widowed, retired accountant with a history of chronic obstructive pulmonary disease was pressured by his only child, a daughter who lives in another state, to be evaluated by a geropsychologist because "he just hasn't been the same" since his wife died 9 months ago. The resident does not think he needs help, and the administrator of the retirement community agrees; he has observed that as one gets frail and has major medical problems, depression is to be expected.

On the other hand, the resident's primary care physician told the resident that if he continued to have problems with eating and sleeping, she would prescribe medication. During the initial consultation with the geropsychologist, the resident's daughter said she thought that it would be better first for her father to talk about his grief over the death of his wife of 40 years, and she was particularly concerned that if her father's functioning continued to deteriorate he might need to be transferred to a higher level of care in a setting where mental health treatment was scarce.

When the geropsychologist interviews the resident, he discovers that the latter has lost 40 pounds since the death of his wife, has little appetite, poor sleep, and has particular trouble enjoying his hobbies of poker and watching sports on TV. More alarmingly, the resident admits that he wishes that he were dead and that he has fleeting suicidal ideation. The geropsychologist talks with the resident about the need for immediate intervention and recommends a course of interpersonal psychotherapy for depression. The resident says that he would be amenable to treatment but worries about the significant copayment that his insurance company charges for mental health visits and is concerned whether he could afford it on his fixed income. Indeed, he would have to make arrangements for transportation to the geropsychologist's office, and he worries about this expense and whether he could even arrange it given his lack of energy.

Based on his years of graduate school courses, supervised practica, and experience working with the older adult population, the geropsychologist understands that the resident is depressed, that there are evidence-based treatments for depression in older adults, and that non-evidence-based beliefs about the unsatisfactory nature of life for older adults impedes referral for treatment. He recently became certified in interpersonal therapy (Hinrichsen, 2008) and feels comfortable administering this treatment on a weekly basis. Knowing that the resident lives alone, the geropsychologist obtains the resident's somewhat reluctant consent to keep his daughter informed about the progress of the treatment. He also obtains consent to talk with one of the resident's old poker buddies and to ask him to check up on him on a daily basis, contracts with the resident to alert him in case he become suicidal, and gives the resident both Crisis Hotline and emergency room numbers to call if he has suicidal thoughts. If the geropsychologist becomes uncomfortable with these arrangements at any time while the resident remains in crisis, he decides to consider requesting in-home services to be provided as another way of monitoring the resident's condition. These steps are in keeping with the geropsychologist's understanding that older White males living alone are a high-risk group for suicide and that there is a strong need to support the patient during this difficult period in his life. In general, the geropsychologist does not try to pressure his patients to agree to things for which they are uncomfortable, but in this case he believes that the severity of the suicide threat merits privileging Principle A (Beneficence and Nonmaleficence) over promoting self-determination (Principle E: Respect for People's Rights and Dignity).

Some problems with ongoing treatment immediately occur. Despite the new federal law requiring mental health copayments to be reduced to the levels of medical copayments (Centers for Medicare & Medicaid Services, 2016), the resident's insurance company carrier reports that it has never heard of the rule and requires a larger copayment than the resident felt he could afford. The geropsychologist begins to realize that some of the other residents in the facility may be in similar circumstances and not have their depression thoroughly evaluated with varied therapeutic options explored because of lack of understanding by the administrator and the primary care physician (see Standards 3.09, Cooperation with Other Professionals, and 3.11, Psychological Services Delivered to or Through Organizations) about depression and the availability of affordable and effective interventions. He resolves to offer free educational presentations to the staff and to improve contact with the administrator and primary care physician so that he can informally educate them about what geropsychology has to offer the residents.

ETHICAL DECISION-MAKING PROCESS

As illustrated in Exhibits 3.1 and 3.2, a sequence of ethical decision-making questions and steps provides a structured approach to addressing ethical challenges. Asking oneself the questions and following the steps for each case is likely to help achieve good outcomes.

Ethical Issues, Tensions, and Resources

When considering how to resolve the ethical challenges, the geropsychologist consulted a variety of professional resources, including the Ethics Code, other guidelines (e.g., *Guidelines for Psychological Practice With Older Adults*, APA, 2014c), and multiple scholarly works (Hartman-Stein, 1998, 2006; Karlin & Norris, 2006; Lichtenberg & Hartman-Stein, 1997; Mezey et al., 2002). In his weighing the positives and negatives of strongly encouraging the involvement of a family member and friend, the geropsychologist carefully balances the benefits of promoting beneficence (Principle A) over self-determination (Principle E). By drawing on his attitudinal, knowledge, and experience base with older adults, the geropsychologist's professional behavior was in accordance with the standards of provision of psychological services within one's boundaries of competence (Standard 2.01). He garnered informed consent (Standard 3.10) from the client to discuss matters and make arrangements with his buddies to check up on him. In keeping with the idea of general advocacy for older adults and their families, and consistent with Principle B (Fidelity and Responsibility), which states in part: "Psychologists consult with, refer to, or cooperate with other professionals and institutions to the extent needed to serve the best interests of those with whom they work," the geropsychologist decides to institute a free monthly seminar series geared to the community staff but open to residents as well as the general public regarding "mental health issues in older adults." In keeping with Principle D (Justice), "psychologists recognize that fairness and justice entitle all persons to access to and benefit from the contributions of psychology and to equal quality in the processes, procedures and services being conducted by psychologists," the geropsychologist did what he could to assure that the community administrator would become more sensitive to the mental health needs of his residents and assist his staff in identifying and making referrals for residents who may need professional help. In keeping with Standards 3.09, Cooperation with Other Professionals, and 3.11, Psychological Services Delivered to or Through Organizations, he also paid a visit to the primary care physician and tried to work out a consulting arrangement whereby the administrator could contact the geropsychologist whenever a question arose about a resident's mental health and ask whether a referral was appropriate.

The geropsychologist was torn between promoting the patient's Autonomy (Principle E) and ensuring the patient's safety from potential strong suicidal urges (Principle A). The severity of the threat, especially regarding the risk factors of being an older White male living by himself, forced the geropsychologist to come down on the side of beneficence. However, if and when the suicidal threat recedes, the geropsychologist must reconsider his position and perhaps begin to allot more weight to respect for autonomy in the patient's decision making. The other ethical tension that the geropsychologist was faced with was how to ethically practice within another organization (Standard 3.11, Psychological Services Delivered to or Through Organizations), and how to cooperate with another professional (Standard 3.09, Cooperation with Other Professionals), whom he believed might be operating outside of his scope of competence and potentially harming other nursing home residents by prescribing psychiatric medications when other approaches should at least be tried first. By making *pro bono* educational experiences available to the staff and by providing the primary care physician with an avenue for professional consultation, the geropsychologist appropriately addressed current ethical concerns. Face-to-face talks with the administrator and the primary care physician regarding the specifics of the management of resident mental health issues may be the next step if similar problems continue.

Preferred Course of Action

The geropsychologist immediately called the local insurance company's number, and when no quick answers were forthcoming, he contacted the insurance company's home office and educated them on the law requiring equal copay for psychiatric conditions. The geropsychologist also contacted the retirement community administrator and requested that the facility arrange transportation to assist this long-time resident in continuing with psychological treatment and in maintaining independent living. These behaviors reflected the need to advocate for an individual client's needs as well as to conduct this advocacy at a corporate level to improve business policies, and the efforts were consistent with Principle A (Beneficence and Nonmaleficence) to safeguard "the welfare and rights" of his client.

The geropsychologist had always understood the need for advocacy for older adults in the abstract, but this case broadened his horizons, and he became more involved with APA and professional geropsychological groups to advocate on a national level for more research on effective treatments for older adults (i.e., general advocacy for the mental health of older adults and their families) and to promote the need for the hiring of trained geriatric mental health professionals to provide care in nursing homes and assisted living facilities (i.e., advocacy for changes in institutional policy). He also lobbied for more liberal reimbursement for psychologists to provide not only treatment but also to allow them time for pro bono education on ageist biases (e.g., "Older adults can't change with psychotherapy because they are too set in their ways" or "Older adults prefer medications to psychotherapy")—in other words, he advocated for improved business practice and insurance reimbursement policies.

CONCLUSION

Many opportunities exist for the public promotion of the goals of geropsychology and the needs of those served by geropsychologists. Such advocacy increases the opportunities for, and strengthens the ability of, geropsychologists to provide meaningful and valuable services to older adults. However, care must be taken to ensure that advocacy activities are pursued in an appropriate and responsible manner. Failure to advocate in an ethical manner threatens the success of otherwise important efforts and can compromise public trust in geropsychology, which can have long-term negative effects on advocacy efforts. Geropsychologists who are invested in influencing public policy in an ethical manner can improve the lives of older adults. A commitment to ethical advocacy and awareness of relevant ethical issues, such as those described in this chapter, are essential components of successful advocacy in geropsychology.

AFTERWORD

Geropsychologists serve older adults, and those involved in the lives and care of older adults, in many ways and in diverse settings. Each professional activity offers the opportunity to better understand older adults and improve their lives or maximize their quality of life, either directly or indirectly. This is no small responsibility; it is one that should be undertaken enthusiastically but not lightly. An important part of that responsibility involves understanding the ethical issues inherent in providing a specific service to a unique individual in a particular setting. Part of understanding geriatric ethical issues is being able to anticipate the ethical challenges that may be encountered and being able to avoid or address the challenges. But such ability does not magically appear upon completion of graduate school or a training program.

Many resources exist to inform and educate geropsychologists about appropriate professional behavior. Geropsychologists are often introduced to relevant published resources in the course of their education and training,

http://dx.doi.org/10.1037/0000010-011
Ethical Practice in Geropsychology, by S. S. Bush, R. S. Allen, and V. A. Molinari

and they continue to pursue additional and new ethical and legal resources throughout their careers. Establishing ethical competence while developing clinical competence prepares geropsychologists to provide beneficial services when they enter practice or transition to a new type of practice. The ethical importance of establishing, maintaining, and examining foundational and functional competencies as described in the Pikes Peak model for training in professional geropsychology is reflected throughout this book.

The ethical decision-making process is facilitated through the use of a decision-making model. We propose a six-step model that helps geropsychologists (a) identify and clarify the ethical issue, distinguishing it from clinical, legal, or other professional issues; (b) clarify the relevant stakeholders, their values, goals, and interests, and the obligations owed to each; (c) identify and review or consult ethical, legal, and professional resources; (d) consider their own personal beliefs and values and the potential impact of each on the decision-making process; (e) consider the possible solutions and their consequences; and (f) implement the plan, evaluate the outcome, and revise as needed. When a working knowledge of the steps has been achieved, they can often be conceptually integrated and addressed implicitly, which was an approach taken with many of the vignettes in this book. However, in novel situations or with particularly complex problems, strict adherence to the model is indicated. This model can be of value when exploring any ethical issue or addressing any ethical challenge, samples of which are provided in this book.

As the vignettes revealed, an important aspect of the ethical decision-making process involves gathering additional information. Many problems arise or are difficult to resolve because of a lack of knowledge or experience with some aspect of practice. Geropsychologists who are able to fill that knowledge gap, through written resources or consultation with others, can often readily determine a good course of action. A proactive approach that involves ongoing self-education and formal continuing education is consistent with positive ethics and the pursuit of high standards of ethical practice.

The future of geropsychology is bright. In recent years, the specialty has developed in many important ways. As professions and their specialties develop, their shared values are identified and reflected in professional and ethical guidelines and standards of practice. As the need for qualified clinicians, researchers, administrators, advocates, and other psychologists serving older adults continues and grows, so will the need for ethics education in geropsychology. As the specialty evolves in the context of a changing society, new issues of ethical importance are likely to be identified, and the importance assigned to various ethical issues may shift. Additional position papers from professional organizations and other scholarly publications may be needed to provide guidance to geropsychologists on emerging and changing aspects of practice.

Geropsychologists, like all health care professionals, are likely to continue to encounter greater use of, and reliance on, technology and telecommunications. Each cohort of older adults will be progressively more comfortable and sophisticated with the use of technology. As a result, geropsychologists will need to prepare for increased use and abuse of the technology, and they are likely to encounter technological manifestations of problems of aging. For example, a patient with a frontotemporal dementia may impulsively engage in an online shopping spree, quickly depleting his funds or getting into significant debt, a process that would have taken much longer and been more difficult to accomplish with traditional shopping in the community. When used appropriately, technology can be advantageous for persons with neurological disorders of aging, but the potential exists for significant and rapid negative effects from poor judgment, memory loss, impulsivity, misperception of online stimuli, and similar problems. From an evaluation perspective, cognitive assessment using telehealth technology can be very valuable for elderly persons who are homebound or live in areas with limited access to geropsychology; however, environmental distractions, technology glitches, and other factors can interfere with the ability to obtain valid results using telehealth cognitive assessments. Another possible problem involves the increased availability of self-driving cars: Such cars will likely help prevent older adults from being in collisions, thus prolonging their ability to drive, but cognitively compromised older adults who have a tendency to wander may be able to do so much farther from their home.

A second changing aspect of practice for geropsychologists involves diversity, broadly defined. The racial and cultural composition of the United States continues to change. In some areas, the historically dominant culture has been replaced by a mixture of races and cultures, with a variety of languages. Such diversity has implications for all aspects of geropsychology practice, such as avoidance versus acceptance of needed services; assessment, including use of interpreters and selection of culturally appropriate stimuli and representative norms; involvement of extended family members; preference for nontraditional interventions; and so on. There will very likely be increased openness of lesbian, gay, bisexual, and transgender (LGBT) status in subsequent cohorts. As the stigma continues to decline and more people openly identify as members of the LGBT community, relevant issues will become more common in the individual, couples, and family treatment provided by older adults. Thus, practitioners must understand the ethical issues associated with working with the increasing diverse older adult patient population.

A third practice context in which older adults will be evaluated and treated is the forensic realm, both civil and criminal. There will be increasing numbers of older adults involved in civil litigation related to accidents and requiring decisional capacity evaluations in both civil and criminal contexts, evaluations to determine competency to be executed, and treatment while incarcerated. The need for geropsychologists to provide these services is expected to increase. Because relatively little has been written about forensic geropsychology overall, let alone the ethical aspects of forensic geropsychology, more specific resources and practice guidelines are likely to be of great value to practitioners. Although the application of psychological ethics to geropsychology will continue to evolve in many ways, the three ways described above are particularly noteworthy.

The discussion of geropsychology ethics is a process. It began well before the publication of this book and will continue long after the book goes out of print. We hope that this first book devoted solely to geropsychology ethics will facilitate the discussion of ethical issues, challenges, and decision making among geropsychologists and serve as a building block for future ethics publications that will continue to advance the field. The highest standards of ethical practice are needed; the welfare of our patients is at stake.

REFERENCES

Ackerson, K. S., Brodsky, S. L., & Zapf, P. A. (2005). Judges' and psychologists' assessments of legal and clinical factors in competence for execution. *Psychology, Public Policy, and Law, 11*, 164–193. http://dx.doi.org/10.1037/1076-8971.11.1.164

Administration on Aging. (2001). *Achieving cultural competence: A guidebook for providers of services to older Americans and their families*. Retrieved from http://archive.org/stream/achievingcultura00admi/achievingcultura00admi_djvu.txt

Alexopoulos, G. S., Reynolds, C. F., III, Bruce, M. L., Katz, I. R., Raue, P. J., Mulsant, B. H., . . . the PROSPECT Group. (2009). Reducing suicidal ideation and depression in older primary care patients: 24-month outcomes of the PROSPECT study. *The American Journal of Psychiatry, 166*, 882–890. http://dx.doi.org/10.1176/appi.ajp.2009.08121779

Allen, R. S., Carden, K. D., & Salekin, K. L. (2015). Prison populations. In N. Pachana (Ed.), *The encyclopedia of geropsychology* (pp. 1–7). New Delhi, India: Springer. http://dx.doi.org/10.1007/978-981-287-080-3_163-1

Allen, R. S., Crowther, M. R., & Molinari, V. (2013). Training in clinical geropsychology: Predoctoral programs, professional organizations and certification. *Training and Education in Professional Psychology, 7*, 285–290. http://dx.doi.org/10.1037/a0033749

Allen, R. S., Eichorst, M. K., & Oliver, J. S. (2013). Advance directives: Planning for the end of life. In J. Werth (Ed.), *Counseling clients near the end of life: A practical guide for the mental health professional* (pp. 53–74). New York, NY: Springer.

Allen, R. S., Harris, G. M., Burgio, L. D., Azuero, C. B., Miller, L. A., Shin, H. J., . . . Parmelee, P. (2014). Can senior volunteers deliver reminiscence and creative activity interventions? Results of the legacy intervention family enactment randomized controlled trial. *Journal of Pain and Symptom Management, 48*, 590–601. http://dx.doi.org/10.1016/j.jpainsymman.2013.11.012

Allen, R. S., Noh, H., Beck, L. N., & Smith, L. J. (2016). Caring for individuals near the end of life. In L. D. Burgio, J. E. Gaugler, & M. M. Hilgeman (Eds.), *The spectrum of family caregiving for adults and elders with chronic conditions* (pp. 142–211). Ontario, Canada: Oxford University Press. http://dx.doi.org/10.1093/med:psych/9780199828036.001.0001

Alzheimer's Association. (2004). Research consent for cognitively impaired adults: Recommendations for institutional review boards and investigators. *Alzheimer Disease and Associated Disorders, 18*, 171–175. http://dx.doi.org/10.1097/01.wad.0000137520.23370.56

American Academy of Clinical Neuropsychology. (2001). Policy statement on the presence of third party observers in neuropsychological assessment. *The Clinical Neuropsychologist, 15*, 433–439.

American Bar Association, & American Psychological Association Assessment of Capacity in Older Adults Project Working Group. (2008). *Assessment of older adults with diminished capacity: A handbook for psychologists.* Washington, DC: Authors.

American Bar Association, American Psychological Association, & National College of Probate Judges. (2006). *Judicial determination of capacity of older adults in guardianship proceedings.* Retrieved from http://www.americanbar.org/tools/digitalassetabstract.html/content/dam/aba/migrated/aging/docs/judges_book_5_24.pdf

American Bar Association Commission on Law and Aging, & American Psychological Association. (2005). *Assessment of older adults with diminished capacity: A handbook for lawyers.* Washington, DC: Authors.

American Bar Association Commission on Law and Aging, & American Psychological Association. (2006). *Judicial determination of capacity of older adults in guardianship proceedings: A handbook for judges.* Washington, DC: Authors.

American Educational Research Association, American Psychological Association, & National Council on Measurement in Education. (2014). *Standards for educational and psychological testing.* Washington, DC: American Educational Research Association.

American Geriatric Society Ethics Committee. (2002). *Making treatment decisions for incapacitated elderly patients without advance directives.* Retrieved from http://www.medicine.emory.edu/ger/bibliographies/geriatrics/bibliography68_files/Making_treatment_decisions_for_incapacitated_older_adults.....pdf

American Medical Association. (2009). *A physician's guide to assessing and counseling older drivers* (2nd ed.). Chicago, IL: Author.

American Psychological Association. (1999). Test security: Protecting the integrity of tests. *American Psychologist, 54,* 1078.

American Psychological Association. (2003). Guidelines on multicultural education, training, research, practice, and organizational change for psychologists. *American Psychologist, 58,* 377–402. http://dx.doi.org/10.1037/0003-066X.58.5.377

American Psychological Association. (2004). Guidelines for psychological practice with older adults. *American Psychologist, 59,* 236–260. http://dx.doi.org/10.1037/0003-066X.59.4.236

American Psychological Association. (2006). *Guidelines and principles for accreditation of programs in professional psychology (G&P).* Retrieved from https://www.apa.org/ed/accreditation/about/policies/guiding-principles.pdf

American Psychological Association. (2007). Record keeping guidelines. *American Psychologist, 62,* 993–1004. http://dx.doi.org/10.1037/0003-066X.62.9.993

American Psychological Association. (2010). *Ethical principles of psychologists and code of conduct (2002, Amended June 1, 2010).* Retrieved from http://www.apa.org/ethics/code/index.aspx

American Psychological Association. (2012a). Guidelines for the evaluation of dementia and age-related cognitive change. *American Psychologist, 67,* 1–9.

American Psychological Association. (2012b). Guidelines for psychological practice with lesbian, gay, and bisexual clients. *American Psychologist, 67*, 10–42.

American Psychological Association. (2013). Specialty guidelines for forensic psychology. *American Psychologist, 68*, 7–19. http://dx.doi.org/10.1037/a0029889

American Psychological Association. (2014a). *Family caregiving.* Retrieved from http://www.apa.org/about/gr/issues/cyf/caregiving-facts.aspx

American Psychological Association. (2014b). *Guidelines for clinical supervision in health service psychology.* Retrieved from http://apa.org/about/policy/guidelines-supervision.pdf

American Psychological Association. (2014c). Guidelines for psychological practice with older adults. *American Psychologist, 69*, 34–65. http://dx.doi.org/10.1037/a0035063

American Psychological Association. (2014d). *Guide to advocacy and research.* Retrieved from http://www.apa.org/about/gr/advocacy/index.aspx

American Psychological Association. (2014e). *A psychologist's guide to federal advocacy.* Washington, DC: Author. Retrieved from http://www.apa.org/about/gr/advocacy/federal-guide.pdf

American Psychological Association. (2015). Guidelines for clinical supervision in health service psychology. *American Psychologist, 70*, 33–46.

American Psychological Association Committee on Aging. (2009). *Multicultural competency in geropsychology.* Washington, DC: American Psychological Association.

American Psychological Association Presidential Task Force on Evidence-Based Practice. (2006). Evidence-based practice in psychology. *American Psychologist, 61*, 271–285. http://dx.doi.org/10.1037/0003-066X.61.4.271

American Psychological Association Presidential Task Force on Integrated Health Care for an Aging Population. (2008). *Blueprint for change: Achieving integrated health care for an aging population.* Washington, DC: American Psychological Association.

Americans With Disabilities Act of 1990, 42 U.S.C. ch. 126.

Andersen, B. L., DeRubeis, R. J., Berman, B. S., Gruman, J., Champion, V. L., & Massie, M. J., . . . Rowland, J. H. (2014). Screening, assessment, and care of anxiety ad depressive symptoms in adults with cancer: An American Society of Clinical Oncology guideline adaptation. *Journal of Clinical Oncology, 32*, 1605–1609. http://dx.doi.org/10.1200/JCO.2013.52.4611

Anderson, G., Herbert, R., Zeffiro, T., & Johnson, N. (2010). *Chronic conditions: Making the case for ongoing care.* Princeton, NJ: Robert Wood Johnson Foundation. Retrieved from http://www.rwjf.org/content/dam/farm/reports/reports/2010/rwjf54583

Ardito, R. B., & Rabellino, D. (2011). Therapeutic alliance and outcome of psychotherapy: Historical excursus, measurements, and prospects for research. *Frontiers in Psychology, 2*, 270. http://dx.doi.org/10.3389/fpsyg.2011.00270

Areán, P. A., & Gum, A. M. (2013). Psychologists at the table in health care reform: The case of geropsychology and integrated care. *Professional Psychology: Research and Practice, 44*, 142–149. http://dx.doi.org/10.1037/a0031083

Association of State and Provincial Psychology Boards. (2013). *Code of conduct.* Retrieved from http://c.ymcdn.com/sites/www.asppb.net/resource/resmgr/ Guidelines/Code_of_Conduct_Updated_2013.pdf?hhSearchTerms=%22code+ and+conduct%22

Attix, D. K., Donders, J., Johnson-Greene, D., Grote, C. L., Harris, J. G., & Bauer, R. M. (2007). Disclosure of neuropsychological test data: Official position of Division 40 (Clinical Neuropsychology) of the American Psychological Association, Association of Postdoctoral Programs in Clinical Neuropsychology, and American Academy of Clinical Neuropsychology. *The Clinical Neuropsychologist, 21*, 232–238. http://dx.doi.org/10.1080/13854040601042928

Bailey, F. A., Allen, R. S., Williams, B. R., Goode, P. S., Granstaff, S., Redden, D. T., & Burgio, K. L. (2012). Do-not-resuscitate orders in the last days of life. *Journal of Palliative Medicine, 15*, 751–759. http://dx.doi.org/10.1089/jpm.2011.0321

Baird, K. A., & Rupert, P. A. (1987). Clinical management of confidentiality: A survey of psychologists in seven states. *Professional Psychology: Research and Practice, 18*, 347–352. http://dx.doi.org/10.1037/0735-7028.18.4.347

Balanced Budget Act of 1997, Pub.L. 105–33, 111 Stat. 251 (enacted August 5, 1997).

Ball, K., Berch, D. B., Helmers, K. F., Jobe, J. B., Leveck, M. D., Marsiske, M., . . . for the ACTIVE Study Group. (2002). Effects of cognitive training interventions with older adults: A randomized controlled trial. *JAMA, 288*, 2271–2281. http://dx.doi.org/10.1001/jama.288.18.2271

Baltes, P. B., & Baltes, M. M. (1990). Psychological perspectives on successful aging: The model of selective optimization with compensation. In P. B. Baltes & M. M. Baltes (Eds.), *Successful aging: Perspectives from the behavioral sciences* (pp. 1–34). New York, NY: Cambridge University Press. http://dx.doi.org/10.1017/ CBO9780511665684.003

Barber v. Superior Court, 195 Cal. Rptr. 484, 147 Cal. App. 3d 1006 (1983).

Barnett, J. E., Erickson Cornish, J. A., Goodyear, R. K., & Lichtenberg, J. W. (2007). Commentaries on the ethical and effective practice of clinical supervision. *Professional Psychology: Research and Practice, 38*, 268–275. http://dx.doi. org/10.1037/0735-7028.38.3.268

Bass, B. (1985). *Leadership and performance beyond expectations.* New York, NY: Free Press.

Beauchamp, T. L., & Childress, A. F. (2013). *Principles of biomedical ethics* (7th ed.). New York, NY: Oxford University Press.

Becker, M., & Mehra, S. (2010). *SMI in Florida nursing homes: A study of resident, facility and cost characteristics* (Mental Health Law & Policy Faculty Publications, Paper 519). Retrieved from http://scholarcommons.usf.edu/mhlp_facpub/519

Behnke, S. H., Perlin, M. L., & Bernstein, M. (2003). *The essentials of New York mental health law.* New York, NY: Norton.

Bersoff, D. N. (2013, October). APA should stand up against the death penalty. *APA Monitor, 44*(9), 5. Retrieved from http://apa.org/monitor/2013/10/pc.aspx

Birren, J. E., & Schroots, J. J. F. (2001). The history of geropsychology. In J. E. Birren & K. W. Schaie (Eds.), *Handbook of the psychology of aging* (5th ed., pp. 3–28). San Diego, CA: Academic Press.

Blanks, R., & Pinals, D. A. (2007). Competence to be executed. *Journal of the American Academy of Psychiatry and the Law, 35,* 381–384.

Boerner, K., & Jopp, D. (2007). Improvement/maintenance and reorientation as central features of coping with major life change and loss: Contributions of three life-span theories. *Human Development, 50,* 171–195. http://dx.doi.org/10.1159/000103358

Boulton, G. (2014, August 25). With the aging population, the need for more geriatricians grows. *Milwaukee-Wisconsin Journal Sentinel.* Retrieved from http://www.jsonline.com/business/with-aging-population-need-for-more-geriatricians-grows-b99328377z1-272648951.html

Bowers v. Hardwick, 478 U.S. 186 (1985).

Brandl, B., Dyer, C. B., Jeisler, C. J., Marla, J., Stiegel, L. A., & Thomas, R. W. (2007). *Elder abuse detection and intervention: A collaborative approach.* New York, NY: Springer.

Brophy v. New England Sinai Hospital Inc., 497 NE 2d 626 (1986).

Browndyke, J. N. (2004). Ethical challenges with the use of information technology and telecommunications in neuropsychology, part I. In S. S. Bush (Ed.), *A casebook of ethical challenges in neuropsychology* (pp. 179–189). New York, NY: Psychology Press.

Burgio, L., & Kowalkowski, J. D. (2011). Alive and well: The state of behavioral gerontology in 2011. *Behavior Therapy, 42,* 3–8. http://dx.doi.org/10.1016/j.beth.2010.08.003

Burns, B. J., Wagner, H. R., Taube, J. E., Magaziner, J., Permutt, T., & Landerman, L. R. (1993). Mental health service use by the elderly in nursing homes. *American Journal of Public Health, 83,* 331–337. http://dx.doi.org/10.2105/AJPH.83.3.331

Bush, S. S. (2007). *Ethical decision making in clinical neuropsychology.* New York, NY: Oxford University Press.

Bush, S. S. (2009). *Geriatric mental health ethics: A casebook.* New York, NY: Springer.

Bush, S. S. (2012). Ethical considerations in the psychological evaluation and treatment of older adults. In S. Knapp (Ed.), *APA handbook of ethics in psychology: Vol. II. Practice, teaching, and research* (pp. 15–28). Washington, DC: American Psychological Association. http://dx.doi.org/10.1037/13272-002

Bush, S. S. (2014). Ethical, legal, and professional considerations in the psychological assessment of veterans. In S. S. Bush (Ed.), *Psychological assessment of veterans* (pp. 494–514). New York, NY: Oxford University Press.

Bush, S. S., Allen, R. S., Heck, A. L., & Moye, J. (2015). Ethical issues in geropsychology: Clinical and forensic perspectives. *Psychological Injury and Law, 8,* 348–356. http://dx.doi.org/10.1007/s12207-015-9242-2

Bush, S. S., Connell, M. A., & Denney, R. L. (2006). *Ethical practice in forensic psychology: A systematic model for decision making.* Washington, DC: American Psychological Association. http://dx.doi.org/10.1037/11469-000

Bush, S., & Martin, T. (2004). Intermanual differences on the Rey Complex Figure Test. *Rehabilitation Psychology, 49,* 76–78. http://dx.doi.org/10.1037/0090-5550.49.1.76

Bush, S. S., & Martin, T. A. (2006). The ethical and clinical practice of disclosing raw test data: Addressing the ongoing debate. *Applied Neuropsychology, 13,* 115–124. http://dx.doi.org/10.1207/s15324826an1302_6

Bush, S. S., Rapp, D. L., & Ferber, P. S. (2010). Maximizing test security in forensic neuropsychology. In A. M. Horton, Jr., & L. C. Hartlage (Eds.), *Handbook of forensic neuropsychology* (2nd ed., pp. 177–195). New York, NY: Springer.

Bush, S. S., Ruff, R. M., Tröster, A. I., Barth, J. T., Koffler, S. P., Pliskin, N. H., Reynolds, C. R., & Silver, C. H. (2005). Symptom validity assessment: Practice issues and medical necessity. Official position of the National Academy of Neuropsychology. *Archives of Clinical Neuropsychology, 20,* 419–426.

Butler, R. N. (1963). The life review: An interpretation of reminiscence in the aged. *Psychiatry, 26,* 65–76.

Byrd, D. A., & Manly, J. J. (2012). Cultural considerations in the neuropsychological assessment of older adults. In S. S. Bush & T. A. Martin (Eds.), *Geriatric neuropsychology: Practice essentials* (pp. 115–139). New York, NY: Psychology Press.

Cain, D. J., Keenan, K., & Rubin, S. (Eds.). (2015). *Humanistic psychotherapies: Handbook of research and practice* (2nd ed.). Washington, DC: American Psychological Association.

California Health and Safety Code, Section 103.900. Retrieved from http://www.leginfo.ca.gov/cgi-bin/displaycode?section=hsc&group=103001-104000&file=103900

Camp, C. J., & Lee, M. M. (2011). Montessori-based activities as a transgenerational interface for persons with dementia and preschool children. *Journal of Intergenerational Relationships, 9,* 366–373. http://dx.doi.org/10.1080/15350770.2011.618374

Campbell, L. M., & Amin, N. (2012). A poststructural glimpse at the World Health Organization's palliative care discourse in rural South Africa. *Rural and Remote Health, 12,* 2059–2066.

Canadian Psychological Association. (2000). *Canadian code of ethics for psychologists* (3rd ed.). Ottawa, Ontario, Canada: Author.

Caplan, B., & Shechter, J. (2012). Test accommodations in geriatric neuropsychology. In S. S. Bush & T. A. Martin (Eds.), *Geriatric neuropsychology: Practice essentials* (pp. 97–114). New York, NY: Psychology Press.

Carlson, M. C. (2011). Introduction: A life course perspective on activity and neurocognitive health. *Journal of the International Neuropsychological Society, 17,* 970–974. http://dx.doi.org/10.1017/S1355617711001366

Carpenter, B. D. (2014, August). Co-teaching interprofessional care at the graduate school level. In J. Moye (Chair), *Advancing Sharon Brehm's vision of integrated care for an aging population*. Pre-conference workshop presented at the 122nd Annual Convention of the American Psychological Association, Washington, DC.

Carpenter, B. D., Sakai, E., Karel, M. J., Molinari, V., & Moye, J. (2016). Training for research and teaching in geropsychology: Preparing the next generation of scholars and educators. *Gerontology & Geriatrics Education, 37*(1), 43–61. http://dx.doi.org/10.1080/02701960.2015.1115981

Carson, E. A. (2014). *Prisoners in 2013*. Retrieved from http://www.bjs.gov/content/pub/pdf/p13.pdf

Carstensen, L. L., Isaacowitz, D. M., & Charles, S. T. (1999). Taking time seriously. A theory of socioemotional selectivity. *American Psychologist, 54,* 165–181. http://dx.doi.org/10.1037/0003-066X.54.3.165

Center for International Human Rights at Northwestern University School of Law. (2011). *Death penalty worldwide: Elderly*. Retrieved from http://www.deathpenaltyworldwide.org/elderly.cfm

Centers for Disease Control and Prevention. (2010). *National hospital discharge survey: 2010 table. Average length of stay and days of care—number and rate of discharges by sex and age*. Retrieved from http://www.cdc.gov/nchs/fastats/older-american-health.htm

Centers for Disease Control and Prevention. (2012). *Health disparities*. Retrieved from http://www.cdc.gov/healthyyouth/disparities/index.htm

Centers for Disease Control and Prevention. (2016). *The Tuskegee timeline*. Retrieved from http://www.cdc.gov/tuskegee/timeline.htm

Centers for Medicare & Medicaid Services. (2016). *The Mental Health Parity and Addiction Equity Act of 2008*. Retrieved from https://www.cms.gov/CCIIO/Programs-and-Initiatives/Other-Insurance-Protections/mhpaea_factsheet.html

Charles, S. T. (2010). Strength and vulnerability integration: A model of emotional well-being across adulthood. *Psychological Bulletin, 136,* 1068–1091. http://dx.doi.org/10.1037/a0021232

Chettiar, I. M., Bunting, W., & Schotter, G. (2012). *At America's expense: The mass incarceration of the elderly*. New York, NY: American Civil Liberties Association.

Chiriboga, D. A. (1997). Crisis, challenge, and stability in the middle years. In M. E. Lachman & J. B. James (Eds.), *Multiple paths of midlife development* (pp. 293–322). Chicago, IL: University of Chicago Press.

Chochinov, H. (2012). *Dignity therapy: Final words for final days*. New York, NY: Oxford University Press. http://dx.doi.org/10.1093/acprof:oso/9780195176216.001.0001

Chow, E., Harth, T., Hruby, G., Finkelstein, J., Wu, J., & Danjoux, C. (2001). How accurate are physicians' clinical predictions of survival and the available prognostic tools in estimating survival times in terminally ill cancer patients? A systematic review. *Clinical Oncology, 13,* 209–218.

Christakis, N. A., & Lamont, E. B. (2000). Extent and determinants of error in doctors' prognoses in terminally ill patients: Prospective cohort study. *British Medical Journal, 320*, 469–473. http://dx.doi.org/10.1136/bmj.320.7233.469

Clark, R. A., Harden, S. L., & Johnson, W. B. (2000). Mentor relationships in clinical psychology doctoral training: Results of a national survey. *Teaching of Psychology, 27*, 262–268. http://dx.doi.org/10.1207/S15328023TOP2704_04

Clay, R. (2006). Geropsychology grants in peril: Seven geropsychology training efforts have lost funding they receive through the Federal Graduate Psychology Education (GPE) Program. *Monitor on Psychology, 37*, 46.

Cohen-Mansfield, J., Marx, M. S., Dakheel-Ali, M., & Thein, K. (2015). The use and utility of specific nonpharmacological interventions for behavioral symptoms in dementia: An exploratory study. *The American Journal of Geriatric Psychiatry, 23*, 160–170.

Colenda, C. C., Bartels, S. C., & Gottlieb, G. L. (1999). The North American system of care. In J. Copeland, M. Abou-Saleh, & D. Blazer (Eds.), *Principles and practices of geriatric psychiatry* (2nd ed., pp. 689–696). London, England: Wiley and Sons.

Connors, A. F., Jr., Dawson, N. V., Desbiens, N. A., Fulkerson, W. J., Goldman, L., Knaus, W. A., . . . Ransohoff, D. (1995). A controlled trial to improve care for seriously ill hospitalized patients. The study to understand prognoses and preferences for outcomes and risks of treatments (SUPPORT). *JAMA, 274*, 1591–1598. http://dx.doi.org/10.1001/jama.1995.03530200027032

Council of Professional Geropsychology Training Programs. (2013). *Pikes Peak geropsychology knowledge and assessment tool, version 1.2*. Retrieved from http://copgtp.org/wp-content/uploads/2016/01/Pikes-Peak-Evaluation-Tool-1.4.pdf

Coverdale, J., McCullough, L. B., Molinari, V., & Workman, R. (2006). Ethically justified clinical strategies for promoting geriatric assent. *International Journal of Geriatric Psychiatry, 21*, 151–157. http://dx.doi.org/10.1002/gps.1443

Crain, W. (2011). *Theories of development: Concepts and applications* (6th ed.). Boston, MA: Pearson Education Inc./Prentice Hall.

Cruzan v. Director, Missouri Department of Health, 497 U.S. 261, 279 (1990).

Davitt, J. K., & Gellis, Z. D. (2011). Integrating mental health parity for homebound older adults under the Medicare home health care benefit. *Journal of Gerontological Social Work, 54*, 309–324. http://dx.doi.org/10.1080/01634372.2010.540075

Death with dignity around the US. (2016, May 24). *Death with Dignity*. Retrieved from https://www.deathwithdignity.org/take-action/

Demakis, G. J. (2012). Looking ahead: Directions for future research in civil capacities. In G. J. Demakis (Ed.), *Civil capacities in clinical neuropsychology: Research findings and practical applications* (pp. 310–316). New York, NY: Oxford University Press.

Donders, J., & Kirkwood, M. W. (2013). Symptom validity assessment with special populations. In D. A. Carone & S. S. Bush (Eds.), *Mild traumatic brain injury: Symptom validity assessment and malingering* (pp. 399–410). New York, NY: Springer.

Doukas, D. J., & McCullough, L. B. (1991). The values history. The evaluation of the patient's values and advance directives. *The Journal of Family Practice, 32*, 145–153.

Dziak, K., Anderson, R., Sevick, M. A., Weisman, C. S., Levine, D. W., & Scholle, S. H. (2005). Variations among Institutional Review Board reviews in a multi-site health services research study. *Health Services Research, 40*, 279–290. http://dx.doi.org/10.1111/j.1475-6773.2005.00353.x

Edelstein, B., & Koven, L. (2011). Older adult assessment issues and strategies. In V. Molinari (Ed.), *Specialty competencies in geropsychology* (pp. 41–57). New York, NY: Oxford University Press.

Edelstein, B. A., Woodhead, E. L., Segal, D., Heisel, M. J., Bower, E. H., Lowery, A. J., & Stoner, S. A. (2008). Older adult psychological assessment: Current instrument status and related considerations. *Clinical Gerontologist, 31*, 1–35. http://dx.doi.org/10.1080/07317110802072108

Egan, E. (2012). *VA home based primary care program: A primer and lessons.* Retrieved from http://americanactionforum.org/sites/default/files/VA%20HBPC%20Primer%20FINAL.pdf

Eisenstadt v. Baird, 405 U.S. 438 (1972).

Elder, G. H., Jr. (1985). Perspectives on the life course. In G. H. Elder, Jr. (Ed.), *Life course dynamics* (pp. 23–49). Ithaca, NY: Cornell University Press.

Elder, G. H., Jr. (1998). The life course as developmental theory. *Child Development, 69*, 1–12. http://dx.doi.org/10.1111/j.1467-8624.1998.tb06128.x

Elder, G. H., Jr., Johnson, K. M., & Crosnoe, R. (2003). The emergence and development of life course theory. In J. T. Mortimer & M. J. Shanahan (Eds.), *Handbook of the life course* (pp. 3–19). Hingham, MA: Kluwer Academic. http://dx.doi.org/10.1007/978-0-306-48247-2_1

Emery, E. E. (2011). Integrative care models. In V. Molinari (Ed.), *Specialty competencies in geropsychology* (pp. 84–100). New York, NY: Oxford University Press.

Engel, J., & Prentice, D. (2013). The ethics of interprofessional collaboration. *Nursing Ethics, 20*, 426–435. http://dx.doi.org/10.1177/0969733012468466

Erikson, E. H. (1950). *Childhood and society.* New York, NY: Norton.

Falender, C. A., & Shafranske, E. P. (2004). *Clinical supervision: A competency-based approach.* Washington, DC: American Psychological Association. http://dx.doi.org/10.1037/10806-000

Falender, C. A., & Shafranske, E. P. (2007). Competence in competency-based supervision practice: Construct and application. *Professional Psychology: Research and Practice, 38*, 232–240. http://dx.doi.org/10.1037/0735-7028.38.3.232

Falender, C. A., & Shafranske, E. P. (2013, March/April). Clinical supervision and risk management. *The California Psychologist*, 9–11.

Family Caregiver Alliance. (2001). *Dementia, driving and California state law*. Retrieved from https://www.caregiver.org/dementia-driving-and-california-state-law

Family Protection and Domestic Violence Intervention Act of 1994, CRI 831-4 FAMPD 99-721 (1997).

Federal Bureau of Prisons. (2016a). *Inmate age*. Retrieved from https://www.bop.gov/about/statistics/statistics_inmate_age.jsp

Federal Bureau of Prisons. (2016b). *Inmate race*. Retrieved from http://www.bop.gov/about/statistics/statistics_inmate_race.jsp

Feinsod, F. M., & Wagner, C. (2007). 10 ethical principles in Geriatrics and long-term care. *Annals of Long Term Care, 15*, 24.

Fernandez-Ballesteros, R., Marquez-Gonzalez, M. O., & Santacreu, M. (2014). Geropsychological assessment. In N. A. Pachana & K. Laidlaw (Eds.), *The Oxford Handbook of clinical geropsychology* (pp. 184–222). New York, NY: Oxford University Press.

Fishel, D. (Director). (2004). *Still doing it: The intimate lives of women over 65* [Video]. Blooming Grove, NY: New Day Films.

Fisher, C. B. (2012). Human rights and psychologists' involvement in assessments related to death penalty cases. *Ethics & Behavior, 23*, 58–61. http://dx.doi.org/10.1080/10508422.2013.749761

Fisher, C. B. (2013). *Are psychologists violating their Ethics Code by conducting death penalty evaluations for defendants with mental disabilities?* Retrieved from http://ethicsandsociety.org/2013/05/17/are-psychologists-violating-the-american-psychological-associations-apa-ethics-code-when-they-conduct-death-penalty-evaluations-involving-defendants-with-mental-disabilities/

Fisher, J. M., Johnson-Greene, D., & Barth, J. T. (2002). Examination, diagnosis, and interventions in clinical neuropsychology in general and with special populations: An overview. In S. S. Bush & M. L. Drexler (Eds.), *Ethical issues in clinical neuropsychology* (pp. 3–22). Lisse, Netherlands: Swets & Zeitlinger.

Ford v. Wainwright, 477 U.S. 399, 106 S. Ct. 2595 (1986).

Fouad, H. A., Grus, C. L., Hatcher, R. L., Kaslow, N. J., Smith Hutchings, P., . . . Crossman, R. E. (2009). Competency benchmarks: A model for understanding and measuring competence in professional psychology across training levels. *Training and Education in Professional Psychology, 3* (4, Suppl.), S5–S26.

France, C. R., Masters, K. S., Belar, C. D., Kerns, R. D., Klonoff, E. A., Larkin, K. T., . . . Thorn, B. E. (2008). Application of the competency model to clinical health psychology. *Professional Psychology: Research and Practice, 39*, 573–580. http://dx.doi.org/10.1037/0735-7028.39.6.573

Gatz, M. (2007). Commentary on evidence-based psychological treatments for older adults. *Psychology and Aging, 22*, 52–55. http://dx.doi.org/10.1037/0882-7974.22.1.52

Gelso, C. J. (2006). On the making of a scientist–practitioner: A theory of research training in professional psychology. *Training and Education in Professional Psychology, S*(1), 3–16. http://dx.doi.org/10.1037/1931-3918.S.1.3

Gert, B., Culver, C. M., & Clouser, K. D. (2006). *Bioethics: A systematic approach.* New York, NY: Oxford University Press. http://dx.doi.org/10.1093/0195159063.001.0001

Giele, J. Z., & Elder, G. H. (Eds.). (1998). *Methods of life course research: Qualitative and quantitative approaches.* Thousand Oaks, CA: Sage.

Gordon, B. H., & Karel, M. J. (2014). Psychological assessment of veterans in home based primary care. In S. S. Bush (Ed.), *Psychological assessment of veterans* (pp. 127–158). New York, NY: Oxford University Press.

Griswold v. Connecticut, 381 U.S. 479 (1965).

Guilmette, T. J. (2013). The role of clinical judgment in symptom validity assessment. In D. A. Carone & S. S. Bush (Eds.), *Mild traumatic brain injury: Symptom validity assessment and malingering* (pp. 31–43). New York, NY: Springer.

Guo, Y., Palmer, J. L., Bianty, J., Konzen, B., Shin, K., & Bruera, E. (2010). Advance directives and do-not-resuscitate orders in patients with cancer with metastatic spinal cord compression: Advanced care planning implications. *Journal of Palliative Medicine, 13,* 513–517. http://dx.doi.org/10.1089/jpm.2009.0376

Haber, D. (2006). Life review: Implementation, theory, research, and therapy. *International Journal of Aging and Human Development, 62,* 153–171.

Haley, W. E., Larson, D. G., Kasl-Godley, J., Neimeyer, R. A., & Kwilosz, D. M. (2003). Roles for psychologists in end-of-life care: Emerging models of practice. *Professional Psychology: Research and Practice, 34,* 626–633. http://dx.doi.org/10.1037/0735-7028.34.6.626

Hanson, S. L., Kerkhoff, T. R., & Bush, S. S. (2005). *Health care ethics for psychologists: A casebook.* Washington, DC: American Psychological Association. http://dx.doi.org/10.1037/10845-000

Hartman-Stein, P. E. (1998). Hope amidst the behavioral healthcare crisis. In P. Hartman-Stein (Ed.), *Innovative behavioral healthcare for older adults: A guidebook for changing times* (pp. 201–214). San Francisco, CA: Jossey-Bass.

Hartman-Stein, P. E. (2006). The basics of building and managing a geropsychology practice. In S. H. Qualls & B. G. Knight (Eds.), *Psychotherapy for depression in older adults* (pp. 229–249). Hoboken, NJ: John Wiley & Sons.

Hartman-Stein, P. E., & Ergun, M. (1998). Marketing strategies for geriatric behavioral healthcare. In P. Hartman-Stein (Ed.), *Innovative behavioral healthcare for older adults: A guidebook for changing times* (pp. 179–199). San Francisco, CA: Jossey-Bass.

Hartman-Stein, P. E., & Georgoulakis, J. M. (2008). How Medicare shapes behavioral health practice in older adults in the US: Issues and recommendations for practitioners. In D. Gallagher-Thompson, A. M. Steffen, & L. W. Thompson (Eds.), *Handbook of behavioral and cognitive therapies with older adults* (pp. 323–334). New York, NY: Springer. http://dx.doi.org/10.1007/978-0-387-72007-4_21

Hathaway, S. R., & McKinley, J. C. (1943). *Minnesota Multiphasic Personality Inventory.* Minneapolis: University of Minnesota.

Haut, M. W., & Muehleman, T. (1986). Informed consent: The effects of clarity and specificity on disclosure in a clinical interview. *Psychotherapy: Theory, Research, Practice, Training, 23,* 93–101. http://dx.doi.org/10.1037/h0085598

Hawaii Psychiatric Society v. Ariyoshi, 481 F. Supp. 1028 (D. Hawaii, 1979).

Hays, J. R. (1999). Ethics of treatment in geropsychology: Status and challenges. In M. Duffy (Ed.), *Handbook of counseling and psychotherapy with older adults* (pp. 662–676). New York, NY: John Wiley & Sons.

Hays, J. R., & Jennings, F. L. (2015). Ethics in geropsychology: Status and challenges. In P. Lichtenberg & B. Mast (Eds.), *APA handbook of clinical geropsychology* (pp. 177–192). Washington, DC: American Psychological Association.

Health Care Financing Administration. (1992). Medicare and Medicaid programs: Preadmission screening and annual resident review. *Federal Register, 57*, 56450–56504.

Health Insurance Portability and Accountability Act of 1996, Pub.L. 104–191, 110 Stat. 1936.

Heaton, R. K., Chelune, G. J., Talley, J. L., Kay, G. G., & Curtiss, G. (1993). *Wisconsin Card Sorting Test Manual: Revised and expanded.* Lutz, FL: Psychological Assessment Resources.

Heckhausen, J., & Schulz, R. (1995). A life-span theory of control. *Psychological Review, 102*, 284–304. http://dx.doi.org/10.1037/0033-295X.102.2.284

Heckhausen, J., Wrosch, C., & Schulz, R. (2010). A motivational theory of life-span development. *Psychological Review, 117*, 32–60. http://dx.doi.org/10.1037/a0017668

Heilbronner, R. L., Sweet, J. J., Morgan, J. E., Larrabee, G. J., Millis, S. R., & the Conference Participants. (2009). American Academy of Clinical Neuropsychology Consensus Conference Statement on the neuropsychological assessment of effort, response bias, and malingering. *The Clinical Neuropsychologist, 23*, 1093–1129. http://dx.doi.org/10.1080/13854040903155063

Hinrichsen, G. A. (2006). Why multicultural issues matter for practitioners working with older adults. *Professional Psychology: Research and Practice, 37*, 29–35. http://dx.doi.org/10.1037/0735-7028.37.1.29

Hinrichsen, G. A. (2008). Interpersonal psychotherapy for late life depression: Current status and new applications. *Journal of Rational-Emotive & Cognitive-Behavior Therapy, 26*, 263–275. http://dx.doi.org/10.1007/s10942-008-0086-5

Hinrichsen, G. A. (2011). Interpersonal psychotherapy and psychodynamic psychotherapy. In V. Molinari (Ed.), *Specialty competencies in geropsychology* (pp. 58–66). New York, NY: Oxford University Press.

Hinrichsen, G. A., Kietzman, K. G., Alkema, G. E., Bragg, E. J., Hensel, B. K., Miles, T. P., . . . Zerzan, J. (2010). Influencing public policy to improve the lives of older Americans. *The Gerontologist, 50*, 735–743. http://dx.doi.org/10.1093/geront/gnq034

Hinrichsen, G. A., Zeiss, A. M., Karel, M. J., & Molinari, V. A. (2010). Competency-based geropsychology training in doctoral internships and postdoctoral fellowships. *Training and Education in Professional Psychology, 4*, 91–98. http://dx.doi.org/10.1037/a0018149

Hitov, S. A. (1974). Transfer trauma: Its impact on the elderly. *Clearinghouse Review, 8,* 846.

Hoge, M. A., Karel, M. J., Zeiss, A. M., Alegria, M., & Moye, J. (2015). Strengthening psychology's workforce for older adults: Implications of the Institute of Medicine's report to congress. *American Psychologist, 70,* 265–278.

Holloway, E. L. (1992). Supervision: A way of learning and teaching. In S. D. Brown & R. W. Lent (Eds.), *Handbook of counseling psychology* (2nd ed., pp. 177–214). New York, NY: Wiley.

Hunkeler, E. M., Katon, W., Tang, L., Williams, J. W., Jr., Kroenke, K., Lin, E. H. B., . . . Unützer, J. (2006). Long term outcomes from the IMPACT randomised trial for depressed elderly patients in primary care. *British Medical Journal, 332,* 259–263. http://dx.doi.org/10.1136/bmj.38683.710255.BE

Institute of Medicine. (2012). *The mental health and substance use workforce for older adults: In whose hands?* Washington, DC: National Academies Press.

Interprofessional Education Collaborative. (2016). *Resources.* Retrieved from https://ipecollaborative.org/Resources.html

Israel, B. A., Coombe, C. M., Cheezum, R. R., Schulz, A. J., McGranaghan, R. J., Lichtenstein, R., . . . Burris, A. (2010). Community-based participatory research: A capacity-building approach for policy advocacy aimed at eliminating health disparities. *American Journal of Public Health, 100,* 2094–2102. http://dx.doi.org/10.2105/AJPH.2009.170506

Israel, B. A., Schulz, A. J., Parker, E. A., & Becker, A. B. (1998). Review of community-based research: Assessing partnership approaches to improve public health. *Annual Review of Public Health, 19,* 173–202. http://dx.doi.org/10.1146/annurev.publhealth.19.1.173

Iwasaki, M., Tazeau, Y. N., Kimmel, D., Baker, N. L., & McCallum, T. J. (2009). Gerodiversity and social justice: Voices of minority elders. In J. L. Chin (Ed.), *Diversity in mind and action: Vol. 3. Social, psychological, and political challenges* (pp. 71–90). Westport, CT: Praeger.

James, B. D., Wilson, R. S., Barnes, L. L., & Bennett, D. A. (2011). Late-life social activity and cognitive decline in old age. *Journal of the International Neuropsychological Society, 17,* 998–1005. http://dx.doi.org/10.1017/S1355617711000531

Jang, Y., Kim, G., Chiriboga, D., & King-Kallimanis, B. (2007). A bidimensional model of acculturation for Korean American older adults. *Journal of Aging Studies, 21,* 267–275. http://dx.doi.org/10.1016/j.jaging.2006.10.004

Johnson-Greene, D., & the NAN Policy & Planning Committee. (2005). Informed consent in clinical neuropsychology practice. Official statement of the National Academy of Neuropsychology. *Archives of Clinical Neuropsychology, 20,* 335–340. http://dx.doi.org/10.1016/j.acn.2004.08.003

Kapp, M. B. (2001). *Lessons in law and aging.* New York, NY: Springer.

Karel, M. J. (2011). Ethics. In V. Molinari (Ed.), *Specialty competencies in geropsychology* (pp. 115–143). New York, NY: Oxford University Press.

Karel, M. J., Emery, E. E., Molinari, V., & the CoPGTP Task Force on the Assessment of Geropsychology Competencies. (2010). Development of a tool to evaluate geropsychology knowledge and skill competencies. *International Psychogeriatrics*, 22, 886–896. http://dx.doi.org/10.1017/S1041610209991736

Karel, M. J., Gatz, M., & Smyer, M. A. (2012). Aging and mental health in the decade ahead: What psychologists need to know. *American Psychologist*, 67, 184–198. http://dx.doi.org/10.1037/a0025393

Karel, M. J., Holley, C., Whitbourne, S. K., Segal, D. L., Tazeau, Y., Emery, E. E., . . . Zweig, R. (2012). Preliminary validation of a tool to assess competencies for professional geropsychology practice. *Professional Psychology: Research and Practice*, 43, 110–117. http://dx.doi.org/10.1037/a0025788

Karel, M. J., Knight, B. G., Duffy, M., Hinrichsen, G. A., & Zeiss, A. M. (2010). Attitude, knowledge and skill competencies for practice in professional geropsychology: Implications for training and building a geropsychology workforce. *Training and Education in Professional Psychology*, 4, 75–84. http://dx.doi.org/10.1037/a0018372

Karel, M. J., Molinari, V., Emery-Tiburcio, E. E., & Knight, B. G. (2015). Pikes Peak conference and competency-based training in professional geropsychology. In P. Lichtenberg & B. Mast (Eds.), *APA handbook of clinical geropsychology* (Vol. I, pp. 19–43). Washington, DC: American Psychological Association. http://dx.doi.org/10.1037/14458-003

Karel, M., Sakai, E., Molinari, V., Moye, J., & Carpenter, B. (2016). Training for geropsychology supervision and practice: Perspectives of geropsychology program graduates. *Training and Education in Professional Psychology*, 10, 37–44. http://dx.doi.org/10.1037/tep0000101

Karlin, B. E., & Karel, M. J. (2014). National integration of mental health providers in VA home-based primary care: An innovative model for mental health care delivery with older adults. *The Gerontologist*, 54, 868–879. http://dx.doi.org/10.1093/geront/gnt142

Karlin, B. E., & Norris, M. P. (2006). Public mental health care utilization by older adults. *Administration and Policy in Mental Health and Mental Health Services Research*, 33, 730–736. http://dx.doi.org/10.1007/s10488-005-0003-5

Karlin, B. E., Visnic, S., Shealy McGee, J., & Teri, L. (2014). Results from the multisite implementation of STAR-VA: A multicomponent psychosocial intervention for managing challenging dementia-related behaviors of veterans. *Psychological Services*, 11, 200–208. http://dx.doi.org/10.1037/a0033683

Kasl-Godley, J. E., King, D. A., & Quill, T. E. (2014). Opportunities for psychologists in palliative care: Working with patients and families across the disease continuum. *American Psychologist*, 69, 364–376. http://dx.doi.org/10.1037/a0036735

Kaslow, N. J., Rubin, N. J., Bebeau, M. J., Leigh, I. W., Lichtenberg, J. W., Nelson, P. D., . . . Smith, I. L. (2007). Guiding principles and recommendations for the assessment of competence. *Professional Psychology: Research and Practice*, 38, 441–451. http://dx.doi.org/10.1037/0735-7028.38.5.441

Kaufman, A. S., & Kaufman, N. L. (2006). *Essentials of clinical supervision.* Hoboken, NJ: John Wiley & Sons.

Kearney, M. H. (2014). Who owns a dissertation, and why does it matter? *Research in Nursing and Health, 37,* 261–264. http://dx.doi.org/10.1002/nur.21611

Kemper, S., & Harden, T. (1999). Experimentally disentangling what's beneficial about elderspeak from what's not. *Psychology and Aging, 14,* 656–670. http://dx.doi.org/10.1037/0882-7974.14.4.656

Kerkhoff, T. R., & Hanson, S. L. (2015). Applied ethics: Have we lost a crucial opportunity? *Rehabilitation Psychology, 60,* 376–378. http://dx.doi.org/10.1037/rep0000067

Kim, G., Parton, J. M., DeCoster, J., Bryant, A. N., Ford, K. L., & Parmelee, P. A. (2013). Regional variation of racial disparities in mental health service use among older adults. *The Gerontologist, 53,* 618–626. http://dx.doi.org/10.1093/geront/gns107

Knapp, S., Gottlieb, M., Berman, J., & Handelsman, M. M. (2007). When laws and ethics collide: What should psychologists do? *Professional Psychology: Research and Practice, 38,* 54–59. http://dx.doi.org/10.1037/0735-7028.38.1.54

Knapp, S. J., Gottlieb, M. C., & Handelsman, M. M. (2015). *Ethical dilemmas in psychotherapy: Positive approaches to decision making.* Washington, DC: American Psychological Association. http://dx.doi.org/10.1037/14670-000

Knapp, S., & VandeCreek, L. (2003). *A guide to the 2002 revision of the American Psychological Association's Ethics Code.* Sarasota, FL: Professional Resource Press.

Knapp, S., & VandeCreek, L. (2005). Ethical and patient management issues with older, impaired drivers. *Professional Psychology: Research and Practice, 36,* 197–202.

Knapp, S., & VandeCreek, L. (2006). *Practical ethics for psychologists: A positive approach.* Washington, DC: American Psychological Association. http://dx.doi.org/10.1037/11331-000

Knapp, S. J., & VandeCreek, L. D. (2012). *Practical ethics for psychologists: A positive approach* (2nd ed.). Washington, DC: American Psychological Association.

Knight, B. G. (2004). *Psychotherapy with older adults* (3rd ed.). Thousand Oaks, CA: Sage. http://dx.doi.org/10.4135/9781452204574

Knight, B. G. (2010). Clinical supervision for psychotherapy with older adults. In N. Pachana, K. Laidlaw, & B. G. Knight (Eds.), *Casebook of clinical geropsychology: International perspectives on practice* (pp. 107–118). Oxford, England: Oxford University Press. http://dx.doi.org/10.1093/med/9780199583553.003.0007

Knight, B. G., Karel, M. J., Hinrichsen, G. A., Qualls, S. H., & Duffy, M. (2009). Pikes Peak model for training in professional geropsychology. *American Psychologist, 64,* 205–214. http://dx.doi.org/10.1037/a0015059

Knight, B. G., & Lee, L. O. (2008). Contextual adult lifespan theory for adapting psychotherapy. In K. Laidlaw & B. Knight (Eds.), *Handbook of emotional disorders in later life: Assessment and treatment* (pp. 59–88). New York, NY: Oxford University Press. http://dx.doi.org/10.1093/med:psych/9780198569459.003.0003

Koocher, G. P., & Keith-Spiegel, P. (1998). *Ethics in psychology: Professional standards and cases.* New York: Oxford University Press.

Lachs, M. S., & Pillemer, K. (2004). Elder abuse. *The Lancet, 364,* 1263–1272. http://dx.doi.org/10.1016/S0140-6736(04)17144-4

Lawton, M. P. (1983). Environment and other determinants of well-being in older people. *The Gerontologist, 23,* 349–357. http://dx.doi.org/10.1093/geront/23.4.349

Lengenfelder, J., & DeLuca, J. (2005). Selection and use of screening measures in geriatric neuropsychology. In S. S. Bush & T. A. Martin (Eds.), *Geriatric neuropsychology: Practice essentials* (pp. 21–39). New York, NY: Taylor and Francis.

Levey, S. M. B., Miller, B. F., & deGruy, F. V., III. (2012). Behavioral health integration: An essential element of population-based healthcare redesign. *Translational Behavioral Medicine, 2,* 364–371. http://dx.doi.org/10.1007/s13142-012-0152-5

Levitan, A. B. (1979). Nursing home dilemma-transfer trauma and the noninstitutional option: A review of the literature. *Clearinghouse Review, 13,* 653.

Lichtenberg, P., & Hartman-Stein, P. E. (1997). Effective geropsychology practice in nursing homes. In L. VandeCreek, S. Knapp, & T. L. Jackson (Eds.), *Innovations in clinical practice: A source book* (Vol. 15, pp. 265–281). Sarasota, FL: Professional Resource Press.

Lichtenberg, P. A., Smith, M., Frazer, D., Molinari, V., Rosowsky, E., Crose, R., . . . Gallagher-Thompson, D. (1998). Standards for psychological services in long-term care facilities. *The Gerontologist, 38,* 122–127. http://dx.doi.org/10.1093/geront/38.1.122

Macciocchi, S. N., & Stringer, A. Y. (2001). Assessing risk and harm: The convergence of ethical and empirical considerations. *Archives of Physical Medicine and Rehabilitation, 82*(Suppl. 2), S15–S19. http://dx.doi.org/10.1016/S0003-9993(01)67310-6

Magaziner, J., German, P., Zimmerman, S. I., Hebel, J. R., Burton, L., Gruber-Baldini, A. L., . . . the Epidemiology of Dementia in Nursing Homes Research Group. (2000). The prevalence of dementia in a statewide sample of new nursing home admissions aged 65 and older: Diagnosis by expert panel. *The Gerontologist, 40,* 663–672. http://dx.doi.org/10.1093/geront/40.6.663

Martin, T. A., & Bush, S. S. (2008). Ethical considerations in geriatric neuropsychology. *NeuroRehabilitation, 23,* 447–454.

Mast, B. T. (2011). *Whole person dementia assessment.* Baltimore, MD: Health Professions Press.

Matarazzo, J. D. (1990). Psychological assessment versus psychological testing. Validation from Binet to the school, clinic, and courtroom. *American Psychologist, 45,* 999–1017. http://dx.doi.org/10.1037/0003-066X.45.9.999

Mather, M., & Carstensen, L. L. (2005). Aging and motivated cognition: The positivity effect in attention and memory. *Trends in Cognitive Sciences, 9,* 496–502. http://dx.doi.org/10.1016/j.tics.2005.08.005

McCaffrey, R. J. (Ed.). (2005). Third party observers [Special issue]. *Journal of Forensic Neuropsychology, 4*(2).

McCaffrey, R. J., Lynch, J. K., & Yantz, C. L. (2005). Third party observers: Why all the fuss? [Special issue] *Journal of Forensic Neuropsychology, 4*(2), 1–15. http://dx.doi.org/10.1300/J151v04n02_01

McCullough, L. B., Wilson, N. L., Teasdale, T. A., Kolpakchi, A. L., & Skelly, J. R. (1993). Mapping personal, familial, and professional values in long-term care decisions. *The Gerontologist, 33,* 324–332. http://dx.doi.org/10.1093/geront/33.3.324

McDougall, G. J., Jr., Becker, H., Pituch, K., Acee, T. W., Vaughan, P. W., & Delville, C. L. (2010). The SeniorWISE study: Improving everyday memory in older adults. *Archives of Psychiatric Nursing, 24,* 291–306. http://dx.doi.org/10.1016/j.apnu.2009.11.001

McElroy, H. K., & Prentice-Dunn, S. (2005). Graduate students' perceptions of a teaching of psychology course. *Teaching of Psychology, 32,* 123–125.

Mental illness and the death penalty. (n.d.). *Capitol punishment in context.* Retrieved from http://www.capitalpunishmentincontext.org/issues/mentalillness

Mezey, M. D., Cassel, C. K., Bottrell, M. M., Hyer, K., Howe, J. L., & Fulmer, T. T. (Eds.). (2002). *Ethical patient care: A casebook for geriatric health care teams.* Baltimore, MD: The Johns Hopkins University Press.

Mitchell, R., Parker, V., Giles, M., & Boyle, B. (2014). The ABC of health care team dynamics: Understanding complex affective, behavioral, and cognitive dynamics in interprofessional teams. *Health Care Management Review, 39,* 1–9. http://dx.doi.org/10.1097/HCM.0b013e3182766504

Molinari, V. (1999). Ethical issues in the clinical management of older adults with personality disorder. In E. Rosowsky, L. Abrams, & R. Zweig (Eds.), *Personality disorders in older adults: Emerging issues in diagnosis and treatment* (pp. 275–287). Mahwah, NJ: Erlbaum.

Molinari, V. (2012). Application of the competency model to geropsychology. *Professional Psychology: Research and Practice, 43,* 403–409. http://dx.doi.org/10.1037/a0026548

Moye, J., Marson, D. C., & Edelstein, B. (2013). Assessment of capacity in an aging society. *American Psychologist, 68,* 158–171. http://dx.doi.org/10.1037/a0032159

National Academy of Neuropsychology. (2000). Presence of third party observers during neuropsychological testing: Official statement of the National Academy of Neuropsychology. *Archives of Clinical Neuropsychology, 15,* 379–380.

National Academy of Neuropsychology. (2001). *NAN definition of a clinical neuropsychologist.* Retrieved from https://www.nanonline.org/docs/PAIC/PDFs/NANPositionDefNeuro.pdf

National Academy of Neuropsychology Policy and Planning Committee. (2000). *Handling requests to release test data, recording and/or reproductions of test data. Official statement of the National Academy of Neuropsychology.* Retrieved from https://www.nanonline.org/docs/ResearchandPublications/PositionPapers/Test%20Security%20Appendix%2003.pdf

National Academy of Neuropsychology Policy and Planning Committee. (2003). *Test security: An update. Official statement of the National Academy of Neuropsychology.* Retrieved from https://www.nanonline.org/docs/PAIC/PDFs/NANTestSecurityUpdate.pdf

National Association for Home Care & Hospice. (2010). *Basic statistics about home care: Updated 2010.* Retrieved from http://www.nahc.org/assets/1/7/10HC_Stats.pdf

National Association for Home Care & Hospice. (2015). *About NAHC.* Retrieved from http://www.nahc.org/about/

National Center on Elder Abuse. (1999). *Types of elder abuse in domestic settings.* Washington, DC: Author.

National Center on Elder Abuse. (2005). *Elder abuse prevalence and incidence.* Washington, DC: Author.

NCS Pearson. (2009). *Advanced clinical solutions for WAIS–IV and WMS–IV: Administration and scoring manual.* San Antonio, TX: Author.

Neal, T. M. S. (2010). Choosing the lesser of two evils: A framework for considering the ethics of competence for execution evaluations. *Journal of Forensic Psychology Practice, 10,* 145–157. http://dx.doi.org/10.1080/15228930903446724

Neugarten, B. L. (1972). Personality and the aging process. *The Gerontologist, 12,* 9–15. http://dx.doi.org/10.1093/geront/12.1_Part_1.9

Norris, M. (2008). Policies and reimbursement: Meeting the needs for mental health care in long-term care. In E. Rosowsky, J. Casciani, & M. Arnold (Eds.), *Geropsychology and long-term care: A practitioner's guide* (pp. 1–11). New York, NY: Springer.

Norris, M. P., Molinari, V., & Ogland-Hand, S. (Eds.). (2002). *Emerging trends in psychological practice in long-term care.* Binghamton, NY: Haworth Press.

Nowell, D., & Spruill, J. (1993). If it's not absolutely confidential, will information be disclosed? *Professional Psychology: Research and Practice, 24,* 367–369. http://dx.doi.org/10.1037/0735-7028.24.3.367

Nydegger, R. (2008). Psychologists and hospice: Where we are and where we can be. *Professional Psychology: Research and Practice, 39,* 459–463. http://dx.doi.org/10.1037/0735-7028.39.4.459

Older Americans Act of 1965, 42 U.S.C. ch. 35 §3001 et seq.

Older Americans Act Amendments of 2006, H. Res. 6197, 109th Cong., Pub.L. 109–365.

Older Americans Reauthorization Technical Corrections Act of 2007, Pub.L. 110–19.

Olmstead v. L. C., 527 U.S. 581 (1999).

Omnibus Budget Reconciliation Act of 1987, Title IV, Subtitle C. Nursing Home Reform Act. Pub.L. 100–203, 101 Stat. 1330 (enacted December 22, 1987).

Omnibus Budget Reconciliation Act of 1989, Pub.L. 101–239.

Omnibus Budget Reconciliation Act of 1990, Pub.L. 101–508, 104 Stat. 1388 (enacted November 5, 1990).

O'Shea Carney, C. K., Gum, A. M., & Zeiss, A. M. (2015). Geropsychology in inter-professional teams across different practice settings. In P. Lichtenberg & B. Mast (Eds.), *APA handbook of clinical geropsychology* (Vol. I, pp. 73–99). Washington, DC: American Psychological Association. http://dx.doi.org/10.1037/14458-005

Packard, E. (2007). Polishing those golden years. *APA Monitor, 38,* 34.

Parekh, A. K., & Barton, M. B. (2010). The challenge of multiple comorbidity for the US health care system. *JAMA, 303,* 1303–1304. http://dx.doi.org/10.1001/jama.2010.381

Patient Protection and Affordable Care Act of 2010, Pub.L. No. 111-148, 124 Stat. 119.

Patient Self-Determination Act, Pub.L. No. 101-508 (1991).

Patterson, D. R., & Hanson, S. L. (1995). Joint Division 22 and ACRM guidelines for postdoctoral training in rehabilitation psychology. *Rehabilitation Psychology, 40,* 299–310.

Peake, T. H., Nussbaum, B. D., & Tindell, S. D. (2002). Clinical and counseling super-vision references: Trends and needs. *Psychotherapy: Theory, Research, Practice, Training, 39,* 114–125.

Phillips, L. L., Fisher, S. E., Allen, R. S., & Burgio, L. D. (2004). Mentorship in the University of Alabama Center for Mental Health and Aging. In J. R. Schwar (Ed.), *Mentoring: structure, design, and implementation. The 15th Annual Student Mentoring Conference on Gerontology and Geriatrics: Keynote Address, Sympo-sia and Posters* (pp. 17–23). Athens: The University of Georgia Gerontology Center.

Pope, K., & Bajt, T. R. (1988). When laws and values conflict: A dilemma for psychologists. *American Psychologist, 43,* 828–829. http://dx.doi.org/10.1037/0003-066X.43.10.828

Prentice-Dunn, S. (2006). Supervision of new instructors: Promoting a rewarding first experience in teaching. *Teaching of Psychology, 33,* 45–47.

Prentice-Dunn, S., Payne, K. L., & Ledbetter, J. M. (2006). Improving teaching through video feedback and consultation. In W. Buskist & S. F. Davis (Eds.), *Handbook of the teaching of psychology* (pp. 295–300). Malden, MA: Blackwell. http://dx.doi.org/10.1002/9780470754924.ch50

Qualls, S. H. (2011). The field of geropsychology. In V. Molinari (Ed.), *Specialty com-petencies in geropsychology* (pp. 14–20). New York, NY: Oxford University Press.

Qualls, S. H., Scogin, F., Zweig, R., & Whitbourne, S. K. (2010). Predoctoral train-ing models in professional geropsychology. *Training and Education in Professional Psychology, 4,* 85–90. http://dx.doi.org/10.1037/a0018504

Qualls, S. H., Segal, D. L., Norman, S., Niederehe, G., & Gallagher-Thompson, D. (2002). Psychologists in practice with older adults: Current patterns, sources of training, and need for continuing education. *Professional Psychology: Research and Practice, 33,* 435–442. http://dx.doi.org/10.1037/0735-7028.33.5.435

Randolph, C. (1998). *Repeatable battery for the assessment of neuropsychological status.* San Antonio, TX: The Psychological Corporation.

Reichman, W., Coyne, A., Borson, S., Negrón, A. E., Rovner, B. W., Pelchat, R. J., . . . Hamer, R. M. (1998). Psychiatric consultation in the nursing home: A survey of six states. *American Journal of Geriatric Psychiatry, 6*, 320–327.

Reichman, W. E., Streim, J. E., & Loebel, J. P. (2004). Legal, ethical, and policy issues. In D. G. Blazer, D. C. Steffens, & E. W. Busse (Eds.), *Textbook of geriatric psychiatry* (3rd ed., pp. 515–528). Washington, DC: American Psychiatric Association.

Reitan, R. M., & Wolfson, D. (1985). *The Halstead-Reitan Neuropsychological Test Battery*. Tucson, AZ: Neuropsychology Press.

Richmond, L. L., Morrison, A. B., Chein, J. M., & Olson, I. R. (2011). Working memory training and transfer in older adults. *Psychology and Aging, 26*, 813–822. http://dx.doi.org/10.1037/a0023631

Rickard, H. C., Prentice-Dunn, S., Rogers, R. W., Scogin, F. R., & Lyman, R. D. (1991). Teaching of psychology: A required course for all doctoral students. *Teaching of Psychology, 18*, 235–237. http://dx.doi.org/10.1207/s15328023top1804_10

Rivera, G. (1972). *Willowbrook: A report on how it is and why it doesn't have to be that way*. New York, NY: Random House.

Rivera Mindt, M., Arentoft, A., Coulehan, K., & Byrd, D. (2013). Considerations for the neuropsychological evaluation of older ethnic minority populations. In L. D. Ravdin & H. L. Katzen (Eds.), *Handbook on the neuropsychology of aging and dementia* (pp. 25–41). New York, NY: Springer. http://dx.doi.org/10.1007/978-1-4614-3106-0_3

Rodolfa, E., Bent, R., Eisman, E., Nelson, P., Rehm, L., & Ritchie, P. (2005). A cube model for competency development: Implications for psychology educators and regulators. *Professional Psychology: Research and Practice, 36*, 347–354. http://dx.doi.org/10.1037/0735-7028.36.4.347

Roe v. Wade, 410 U.S. 113 (1973).

Romans, J. S. C., Boswell, D. L., Carlozzi, A. F., & Ferguson, D. B. (1995). Training and supervision practices in clinical, counseling, and school psychology programs. *Professional Psychology: Research and Practice, 26*, 407–412. http://dx.doi.org/10.1037/0735-7028.26.4.407

Rosen, A. L. (2005). *Testimony to the Policy Committee of the White House Conference on Aging. The shortage of an adequately trained geriatric mental health workforce*. Retrieved from http://www.ncmha.org/docs/WHCoAtestimony.pdf

Rosowsky, E., Casciani, J., & Arnold, M. (2008). *Geropsychology and long-term care: A practitioner's guide*. New York, NY: Springer.

Russo, C. A., & Elixhauser, A. (2006). *Statistical brief #6: Hospitalizations in the elderly population, 2003*. Retrieved from http://www.hcup-us.ahrq.gov/reports/statbriefs/sb6.pdf

Saccuzzo, D. (2015). *Liability for failure to supervise adequately: Let the master beware*. Retrieved from http://e-psychologist.org/index.iml?mdl=exam/show_article.mdl&Material_ID=19

Schatz, P. (2004). Ethical challenges with the use of information technology and telecommunications in neuropsychology, part II. In S. S. Bush (Ed.), *A casebook of ethical challenges in neuropsychology* (pp. 190–198). New York, NY: Psychology Press.

Scherrer, J. F., Xian, H., Bucholz, K. K., Eisen, S. A., Lyons, M. J., Goldberg, J., . . . True, W. R. (2003). A twin study of depression symptoms, hypertension, and heart disease in middle-aged men. *Psychosomatic Medicine, 65,* 548–557. http://dx.doi.org/10.1097/01.PSY.0000077507.29863.CB

Schnell, K., Weiss, C. O., Lee, T., Krishnan, J. A., Leff, B., Wolff, J. L., & Boyd, C. (2012). The prevalence of clinically-relevant comorbid conditions in patients with physician-diagnosed COPD: A cross-sectional study using data from NHANES 1999–2008. *BMC Pulmonary Medicine, 12,* 26. http://dx.doi.org/10.1186/1471-2466-12-26

Scogin, F. R., Hanson, A., & Welsh, D. (2003). Self-administered treatment in stepped-care models of depression treatment. *Journal of Clinical Psychology, 59,* 341–349. http://dx.doi.org/10.1002/jclp.10133

Scogin, F., & Presnell, A. (2011). Applying the Pikes Peak model of treatment competency to the use of cognitive-behavioral therapies with older adults. In V. Molinari (Ed.), *Specialty competencies in geropsychology* (pp. 67–83). New York, NY: Oxford University Press.

Scogin, F., & Shah, A. (2006). Screening older adults for depression in primary care settings. *Health Psychology, 25,* 675–677. http://dx.doi.org/10.1037/0278-6133.25.6.675

Scogin, F., Welsh, D., Hanson, A., Stump, J., & Coates, A. (2005). Evidence-based psychotherapies for depression in older adults. *Clinical Psychology: Science and Practice, 12,* 222–237. http://dx.doi.org/10.1093/clipsy.bpi033

Seegert, L. (2013). *Demand for home-based health care expected to rise.* Retrieved from http://healthjournalism.org/blog/2013/11/demand-for-home-based-health-care-expected-to-rise/

Smith-Bell, M., & Winslade, W. J. (1999). Privacy, confidentiality, and privilege in psychotherapeutic relationships. In D. N. Bersoff (Ed.), *Ethical conflicts in psychology* (2nd ed., pp. 149–155). Washington, DC: American Psychological Association. http://dx.doi.org/10.1037/10329-003

Solano, J. P., Gomes, B., & Higginson, I. J. (2006). A comparison of symptom prevalence in far advanced cancer, AIDS, heart disease, chronic obstructive pulmonary disease and renal disease. *Journal of Pain and Symptom Management, 31,* 58–69. http://dx.doi.org/10.1016/j.jpainsymman.2005.06.007

Spragins, W. A., Lorenzetti, D. L., & The Change Foundation. (2008). *Public expectation and patient experience of integration of healthcare: A literature review.* Retrieved from http://www.integrationresources.ca/resources/public-expectation-and-patient-experience-of-integration-of-health-care-a-literature-review

Stiel, S., Bertram, L., Neuhaus, S., Nauck, F., Ostgathe, C., Elsner, F., & Radbruch, L. (2010). Evaluation and comparison of two prognostic scores and the physicians' estimate of survival in terminally ill patients. *Supportive Care in Cancer, 18,* 43–49. http://dx.doi.org/10.1007/s00520-009-0628-0

Stiers, W., & Stucky, K. (2008). A survey of training in rehabilitation psychology practice in the United States and Canada: 2007. *Rehabilitation Psychology, 53,* 536–543. http://dx.doi.org/10.1037/a0013827

Straus, S. E., Johnson, M. O., Marquez, C., & Feldman, M. D. (2013). Characteristics of successful and failed mentoring relationships: A qualitative study across two academic health centers. *Academic Medicine, 88,* 82–89. http://dx.doi.org/10.1097/ACM.0b013e31827647a0

Stucky, K. J., Bush, S., & Donders, J. (2010). Providing effective supervision in clinical neuropsychology. *The Clinical Neuropsychologist, 24,* 737–758. http://dx.doi.org/10.1080/13854046.2010.490788

Sue, D. W. (2008). Multicultural organizational consultation: A social justice perspective. *Consulting Psychology Journal: Practice and Research, 60,* 157–169.

Sutter, E., McPherson, R. H., & Geeseman, R. (2002). Contracting for supervision. *Professional Psychology: Research and Practice, 33,* 495–498. http://dx.doi.org/10.1037/0735-7028.33.5.495

Tarasoff v. Regents of the University of California, 551 P.2d 334 (Cal. 1976).

Taube, D. O., & Elwork, A. (1990). Researching the effects of confidentiality law on patients' self-disclosures. *Professional Psychology: Research and Practice, 21,* 72–75. http://dx.doi.org/10.1037/0735-7028.21.1.72

Tazeau, Y. N. (2011). Individual and cultural diversity considerations in geropsychology. In V. Molinari (Ed.), *Specialty competencies in geropsychology* (pp. 102–114). New York, NY: Oxford University Press. http://dx.doi.org/10.1093/med:psych/9780195385670.003.0008

Testa, M., & West, S. G. (2010). Civil commitment in the United States. *Psychiatry, 7,* 30–40.

Thielke, S., Vannoy, S., & Unützer, J. (2007). Integrating mental health and primary care. *Primary Care: Clinics in Office Practice, 34,* 571–592. http://dx.doi.org/10.1016/j.pop.2007.05.007

Thomas, B., & Skinner, H. (2012). Dissertation to journal article: A systematic approach (Article ID 862135). *Education Research International.* http://dx.doi.org/10.1155/2012/862135

Tinetti, M. E. (2012). The retreat from advanced care planning. *JAMA, 307,* 915–916. http://dx.doi.org/10.1001/jama.2012.229

Tornstam, L. (2005). *Gerotranscendence: A developmental theory of positive aging.* New York, NY: Springer.

Treatment Advocacy Center. (2015). *Improving civil commitment laws and standards.* Retrieved from http://www.treatmentadvocacycenter.org/fixing-the-system/improving-laws-and-standards

Unützer, J., Katon, W. J., Fan, M.-Y., Schoenbaum, M. C., Lin, E. H. B., Della Penna, R. D., & Powers, D. (2008). Long-term cost effects of collaborative care for late-life depression. *The American Journal of Managed Care, 14,* 95–100.

U.S. Department of Health & Human Services. (2003). *Public Law 104-191: Health Insurance Portability and Accountability Act of 1996.* Retrieved from http://www.hhs.gov/ocr/hipaa

U.S. Department of Health & Human Services. (2016a). *Federal policy for the protection of human subjects ("Common Rule").* Retrieved from http://www.hhs.gov/ohrp/regulations-and-policy/regulations/common-rule/index.html#

U.S. Department of Health & Human Services. (2016b). *OHRP expedited review categories (1998).* Retrieved from http://www.hhs.gov/ohrp/regulations-and-policy/guidance/categories-of-research-expedited-review-procedure-1998/index.html

U.S. Department of Health & Human Services, Administration for Community Living, Administration on Aging. (2015). *Affordable Care Act: Opportunities for the aging network.* Retrieved from http://www.aoa.gov/aging_statistics/health_care_reform.aspx

U.S. Department of Health & Human Services, Administration on Aging. (2006). *Public Law 109-365: Older Americans Act Amendments of 2006.* Retrieved from www.aoa.gov/aoa_programs/oaa/oaa_full.asp

U.S. Department of Health & Human Services, Agency for Healthcare Research and Quality. (2014). *Home-based primary care interventions systematic review.* Retrieved from http://effectivehealthcare.ahrq.gov/index.cfm/search-for-guides-reviews-and-reports/?pageaction=displayproduct&productid=2003#9389

U.S. Department of Health & Human Services, Office of the Inspector General. (2001). *Medicare payments for psychiatric services in nursing homes: A follow up.* Retrieved from www.oig.hhs.gov/oei/reports/oei-02-99-00140.pdf

U.S. Department of Justice, Office of Public Affairs. (2015). *National Medicare fraud takedown results in charges against 243 individuals for approximately $712 million in false billing.* Retrieved from http://www.justice.gov/opa/pr/national-medicare-fraud-takedown-results-charges-against-243-individuals-approximately-712

U.S. Department of Veterans Affairs. (2015). *Home based primary care.* Retrieved from http://www.va.gov/geriatrics/guide/longtermcare/home_based_primary_care.asp

Vacha-Haase, T. (2011). Teaching, supervision, and the business of geropsychology. In V. Molinari (Ed.), *Specialty competencies in geropsychology* (pp. 143–162). New York, NY: Oxford University Press. http://dx.doi.org/10.1093/med:psych/9780195385670.003.0010

Vincent, G. K., & Velkoff, V. A. (2010). *The next four decades. The older population in the United States: 2010 to 2050. Current population reports* (pp. 25–1138). Washington, DC: U.S. Census Bureau. Retrieved from http://www.census.gov/prod/2010pubs/p25-1138.pdf

Walker, L. (2014, December 3). Hours before controversial execution of Scott Panetti, court grants stay. *Newsweek.* Retrieved from http://www.newsweek.com/court-grants-stay-hours-controversial-execution-scott-panetti-288947

Washington v. Glucksberg, 117 SC 2258, 2270 (1997).

Wechsler, D. (2008). *Wechsler Adult Intelligence Scale* (4th ed.). San Antonio, TX: NCS Pearson.

Wechsler, D. (2009). *Wechsler Memory Scale* (4th ed.). San Antonio, TX: NCS Pearson.

Weinstock, R., Leong, G. B., & Silva, J. A. (2010). Competence to be executed: An ethical analysis post Panetti. *Behavioral Sciences & the Law, 28,* 690–706. http://dx.doi.org/10.1002/bsl.951

Werth, J., Jr., & Blevins, D. (Eds.). (2006). *Psychosocial issues near the end of life.* Washington, DC: American Psychological Association.

Wethington, E. (2000). Expecting stress: Americans and the midlife crisis. *Motivation and Emotion, 24,* 85–103. http://dx.doi.org/10.1023/A:1005611230993

Whalen v. Roe, 429 U.S. 589 (1976).

Wharton, T., Shah, A., Scogin, F. R., & Allen, R. S. (2013). Evidence to support the Pikes Peak model: The UA Geropsychology Education Program. *Training and Education in Professional Psychology, 7,* 139–144. http://dx.doi.org/10.1037/a0032285

Whitbourne, S. K., & Whitbourne, S. B. (2014). *Adult development & aging: Biopsychosocial perspectives* (5th ed.). Hoboken, NJ: John Wiley & Sons.

Whitlatch, C. J., Feinberg, L. F., & Tucke, S. S. (2005). Measuring the values and preferences for everyday care of persons with cognitive impairment and their family caregivers. *The Gerontologist, 45,* 370–380. http://dx.doi.org/10.1093/geront/45.3.370

Williams, L. (2000). Long-term care after Olmstead v. L. C.: Will the potential of the ADA's integration mandate be achieved? *Journal of Contemporary Health Law Policy, 17,* 205–239.

Willis, S. L., Tennstedt, S. L., Marsiske, M., Ball, K., Elias, J., Koepke, K. M., . . . Wright, E. (2006). Long-term effects of cognitive training on everyday functional outcomes in older adults. *JAMA, 296,* 2805–2814. http://dx.doi.org/10.1001/jama.296.23.2805

Wilper, A. P., Woolhandler, S., Boyd, J. W., Lasser, K. E., McCormick, D., Bor, D. H., & Himmelstein, D. U. (2009). The health and health care of US prisoners: Results of a nationwide survey. *American Journal of Public Health, 99,* 666–672. http://dx.doi.org/10.2105/AJPH.2008.144279

Wilson, R. S., Mendes De Leon, C. F., Barnes, L. L., Schneider, J. A., Bienias, J. L., Evans, D. A., & Bennett, D. A. (2002). Participation in cognitively stimulating activities and risk of incident Alzheimer disease. *JAMA, 287,* 742–748. http://dx.doi.org/10.1001/jama.287.6.742

Wood, M. E., Salekin, K. L., & Allen, R. S. (2014). Punishment and age. In A. Jamieson & A. Moenssens (Eds.), *Wiley encyclopedia of forensic science* (pp. 1–6). Chichester, England: John Wiley & Sons. http://dx.doi.org/10.1002/9780470061589.fsa252.pub3

Woodard, J. L., & Axelrod, B. N. (2012). Neurological batteries for older adults. In S. S. Bush & T. A. Martin (Eds.), *Geriatric neuropsychology: Practice essentials* (pp. 41–84). New York, NY: Psychology Press.

Woodhead, E. L., Emery, E. E., Pachana, N. A., Scott, T. L., Konnert, C. A., & Edelstein, B. A. (2013). Graduate students' geropsychology training opportunities and perceived competence in working with older adults. *Professional Psychology: Research and Practice, 44,* 355–362. http://dx.doi.org/10.1037/a0034632

Woods, K. M., & McNamara, J. R. (1980). Confidentiality: Its effect on interviewee behavior. *Professional Psychology, 11,* 714–721. http://dx.doi.org/10.1037/0735-7028.11.5.714

World Health Organization. (1996). *Cancer pain relief* (2nd ed.). Geneva, Switzerland: Author.

Yang, J. A., Garis, J., Jackson, C., & McClure, R. (2009). Providing psychotherapy to older adults in home: Benefits, challenges, and decision-making guidelines. *Clinical Gerontologist, 32,* 333–346. http://dx.doi.org/10.1080/07317110902896356

Yoder, M. S., & Turner, T. H. (2014). Assessment via telemental health technology. In S. S. Bush (Ed.), *Psychological assessment of veterans* (pp. 159–173). New York, NY: Oxford University Press.

Zeiss, A. M., & Steffen, A. (1996). Interdisciplinary health care teams: The basic unit of geriatric care. In L. L. Carstensen, B. A. Edelstein, & L. Dornbrand (Eds.), *The handbook of clinical geropsychology* (pp. 423–450). Thousand Oaks, CA: Sage.

Zeltzer, B. B., & Kohn, R. (2006). Mental health services for homebound elders from home health nursing agencies and home care agencies. *Psychiatric Services, 57,* 567–569. http://dx.doi.org/10.1176/ps.2006.57.4.567

Zerzan, J. T., Hess, R., Schur, E., Phillips, R. S., & Rigotti, N. (2009). Making the most of mentors: A guide for mentees. *Academic Medicine, 84,* 140–144. http://dx.doi.org/10.1097/ACM.0b013e3181906e8f

Zimmerman, J. A., Fiske, A., & Scogin, F. (2011). Mentoring in clinical geropsychology: Across the stages of professional development. *Educational Gerontology, 37,* 355–369. http://dx.doi.org/10.1080/03601277.2011.553556

Zweig, R. A., Siegel, L., Byrne, K., Passman, V., Hahn, S., Kuslansky, G., . . . Hinrichsen, G. A. (2005). Doctoral clinical geropsychology training in a primary care setting. *Gerontology & Geriatrics Education, 25,* 109–129. http://dx.doi.org/10.1300/J021v25n04_07

INDEX

University of Alabama, 128, 129
U.S. Department of Health and Human Services (HHS), 139–140, 161–163
U.S. Department of Justice, 101
U.S. Supreme Court, 178–180

Vacha-Haase, T., 121
VandeCreek, L., 42, 46, 73
Veterans Affairs (VA)
    as example of integrated health care, 154
    geropsychologists in, 18
    home-based primary care program, 45–46
    institutional review board of, 140
    telemental health used by, 164

Vulnerable patients
    laws protecting, 53
    protection of, in research, 139–144

Wagner, C., 46
West, S. G., 142
Wethington, E., 14
Woodard, J. L., 80
World Health Organization (WHO), 184
Wundt, Wilhelm, 5

Yang, J. A., 163

Zerzan, J. T., 136

ABOUT THE AUTHORS

Shane S. Bush, PhD, ABPP, is a neuropsychologist and member of the American Psychological Association–accredited geropsychology postdoctoral residency program supervisory staff at the Veterans Affairs New York Harbor Healthcare System. He is also director of Long Island Neuropsychology, PC. He is board certified in Geropsychology, Clinical Psychology, Rehabilitation Psychology, and Clinical Neuropsychology. He is a member of the Board of Directors of the American Board of Geropsychology. Dr. Bush is a fellow of the American Psychological Association (Divisions 12, 18, 20, 22, 40, and 42) and a past president and fellow of the National Academy of Neuropsychology. He has published more than 14 books and special journal issues, including *Geriatric Neuropsychology: Practice Essentials* (coedited with Thomas A. Martin) and *Geriatric Mental Health Ethics: A Casebook*. He has also published numerous articles and book chapters related to ethical practice, including the specialty of geropsychology. He has presented on professional ethics at national and international conferences. Dr. Bush is a veteran of both the U.S. Marine Corps and Naval Reserve.

Rebecca S. Allen, PhD, ABPP, is a professor of psychology and has a primary appointment in the Alabama Research Institute on Aging at The University of Alabama. She is an associate editor of *Aging and Mental Health*. Dr. Allen is a fellow of the Behavioral and Social Sciences section of the Gerontological Society of America and the American Psychological Association (Division 20). She is board certified in geropsychology by the American Board of Professional Psychology (ABGERO) and is an ABGERO board member. Dr. Allen's research and clinical interests focus on interventions to reduce the stress of individuals, family, and professional caregivers for older adults with advanced chronic or terminal illness; the dynamics of health care decision making; and practice and training issues, including ethics. She has published on translation of interventions with older adults near the end of life and their caregivers; diversity in advance care planning; end-of-life issues, including civil capacity, behavioral interventions in long-term care; and mental health among aging prisoners. She teaches clinical psychology of aging intervention, lifespan development, geropsychology practicum, and undergraduate statistics.

Victor Molinari, PhD, ABPP, is a professor in the School of Aging Studies at the University of South Florida. Prior to that, he spent more than 17 years as the director of geropsychology for the Houston Veterans Affairs Medical Center. He is board certified in both clinical psychology and geropsychology. He is past chair of the Council of Professional Geropsychology Training Programs and current president of the American Board of Geropsychology. He was a member of American Psychological Association's (APA's) Task Force on Serious Mental Illness and Severe Emotional Disturbance, and he has served on APA's Committee on Aging. He is the past national coordinator for the Psychologists in Long Term Care and past president of APA's Division 12, Section 2 (Clinical Geropsychology). A former member of the National Institute of Health National Advisory Council on Aging, Dr. Molinari is a fellow of APA's Division 20, the American Academy of Clinical Psychology, and the Behavioral and Social Sciences section of The Gerontological Society of America. He was the major preceptor for a federally funded joint University of South Florida/Tampa Veterans Affairs geropsychology postdoctoral fellowship program, and he is the associate editor for long-term care for the interdisciplinary journal *Clinical Gerontologist*. He teaches courses in gerontological counseling, care management of older adults, and disruptive behavior in long-term care settings.